# Melmark

# *Melmark*

# THE HOME
# THAT LOVE BUILT

## MILDRED KRENTEL

**LOIZEAUX BROTHERS**
*Neptune, New Jersey*

MELMARK—THE HOME THAT LOVE BUILT
May 1988

Printed in the United States of America.

A publication of Loizeaux Brothers, Inc. A nonprofit organization devoted to the Lord's work and to the spread of his truth.

Library of Congress Cataloging-in-Publication Data
Krentel, Mildred.
    Melmark—the home that love built/Mildred Krentel.
    p.    cm.
    ISBN 0-87213-472-5
    1. Melmark Home (Institution) 2. Handicapped children—Institutional care—United States. 3. Down syndrome—Patients—United States—Biography. I. Title.
HV889.5.B47K74 1988
362.4'0485'09748—dc 19

Portions of this book appeared originally in *Melissa Comes Home,* published by Moody Press in 1972. This volume is a revised and updated version of the story of the Melmark Home.

# TO MY GRANDCHILDREN

SCOTT ROBERT KRENTEL

MATTHEW RONALD HODGE (DECEASED)

ALISON MARTHA KRENTEL

BRIAN THOMAS HODGE

JONATHAN DAVID KRENTEL

STEPHEN PAUL HODGE

JULIE CHRISTINE KRENTEL

LAURA PATRICIA KRENTEL

BENJAMIN DAVID KRENTEL

JEFFREY STEPHEN KRENTEL

AMY ELIZABETH KRENTEL

*Melmark*

# 1

The next morning when they brought her into my hospital room for her early feeding, I checked her over carefully. Ten fingers, ten toes—the usual mother's routine.

For the life of me, I couldn't figure out who she looked like. Big brother David, now almost twenty-one? Nineteen-year-old Bob? Diane, all of seventeen and almost breathless in anticipation of the birth of her new baby sister? Even thirteen-year-old Steve, our youngest, did not even faintly resemble Melissa.

Studying her small puffy face intently, I frowned. It was then that I noticed a tiny slant in her large saucer-like eyes. Kind of different, I mused, stroking her cheek tenderly. I propped her alongside me, and she collapsed into a small, defenseless heap, like one of those Japanese sleeping dolls.

Quite unbidden, there flashed through my mind the face of a young girl who had attended our church in Greensboro, North Carolina. She had an unusual first name: Geide. I studied my baby again. Melissa looked exactly like Geide. And I shivered from head to foot, for Geide was mentally retarded—a mongoloid!

*Dear God, how could you?*

I lay back on the pillow. Tears welled up from my broken heart to spill from my eyes. When the nurse came in to take Melissa back to the nursery, I could not bring myself to talk to her. Maybe she would think I was asleep. But she did not even seem to notice, as she walked briskly out of the room hugging my day-old baby close to her.

My sobbing was deep. I wept for myself, too old and too tired to even think of having more babies. And I wept for my husband, my love. Oh, surely this would break his heart.

I lay there in bed waiting for the doctor to affirm my inner

9

suspicions. My premonitions sat like lead in me.

One hour crawled by, and then two. It was pure agony. Finally, I heard heavy footsteps down the hall.

*They must stop at my room, or I will simply scream, and they will know then, that I have gone berserk with grief.*

"And how's the new mother this morning?"

It was the voice of my obstetrician. Turning my face away toward the window, I groped for a semblance of outward composure.

"I'm worried about my baby."

"Now, now, why are you worried? Your little girl is just fine. Her face is a little bruised by the way she came into the world, but outside of that . . ."

His kindly voice trailed off. With a gut wrench inside of me, I suddenly realized that he really did not know. He had watched over Melissa's birthing, but from then on her care was within the pediatrician's domain.

I managed a quick smile so that he would hurry away. He left with reassurances tumbling from his mouth.

*Maybe I am a neurotic older mother. After all, forty-two is a ripe old age to be having babies. But I know that something is wrong with my baby. Where is my baby's doctor?*

When at last the pediatrician appeared in the doorway, I wanted none of his polite chitchat. But he wasn't about to engage in pleasantries. He walked past my bed over to the window, and stood there looking out on the parking lot. Again I felt that cold quiver of apprehension.

I blurted out: "What does a mongoloid baby look like?"

Turning to face me, he answered in a deliberately professional manner, seemingly devoid of any emotion. "The term *mongoloid* is not used anymore; the condition is called Down syndrome. The Down syndrome baby has a broad face; the bridge of his nose is flat; the eyes appear to be almond-shaped. These are the facial signs most easily recognized. And then of course there is the single palmar crease in the hand which is quite common, as well as chromosomal tests."

He sounded like a medical journal.

"Tell me, do you suspect my baby of being a . . . a . . .?" my voice trailed off. I could not say the words.

"I am sorry; I truly am. I was simply waiting for the results of a few more tests. But your suspicions have made it easier for me to break the news to you. Yes, your little baby daughter has Down syndrome. This is a chromosomal abnormality that happens at the moment of conception and frequently occurs in babies of older mothers like yourself."

Well, there it was. Although I had been waiting for his verdict, his conclusions caught me off balance. This was a giant pill for me to swallow all by myself.

*Surely my heart is strangling and there is no air for me to breathe. What is happening? Is this what it feels like to die? Who will take care of my handicapped baby? How can I ever teach her? What do I know about all this? Who told me something like this could happen? Who warned me of the hidden dangers that a mother over forty could encounter? Where were all the doctors then?*

Deep down inside me, where no one could see, I was desperately bitter. On the outside, I wore a bleak smile. I really did not want to hear any more of his explanations. I had given birth to a mentally-retarded child. It was a cold, grim fact. Now, I had to weigh the size and shape of this awful thing that had happened. My mind was spinning.

*Go away, please go. Don't try your words of comfort on me, please. I need to be alone.*

But he kept on talking, suggesting that we place Melissa in an institution where she could be trained properly and have friends like herself.

*Surely you must be mad. You're not making sense. If you don't leave soon, you will see me turn inside out right before your very eyes. My turmoil will be laid bare.*

"Thank you," I managed to mumble inanely.

He turned away and walked out of my room, with just a trace of a sad little smile and a helpless, "If there's anything I can do . . ."

There is a spiritual called, "I Won't Have to Cross Jordan Alone." This was a terrifying Jordan, my own personal Jordan, and I needed to get about crossing it. I felt a million miles away from the God who had promised to cross with me. I could not seem to find his hand. It seemed to me, in these first awe-filled moments of knowing, that this time I would have to cross all by myself.

I put in a long-distance phone call for my husband, who had flown to Pittsburgh on business earlier in the morning, just bursting with happiness and pride over our newest baby. He was in the office of one of the vice presidents of United States Steel when I finally reached him.

"Paul . . ." the word hung there, spanning the miles.

"What's wrong, Miggy? Are you OK?"

"It's not me. It's our baby. The doctor just left and he told me . . . Melissa is retarded."

It was a cruel package of words to wrap up a heartache. The impact was immediate.

"I'll be there as soon as I can catch a flight."

He was at my side in two-and-a-half hours. He stood framed in the doorway of my hospital room for a long minute just looking at me. Then he walked solemnly over to my bed and gathered me close while tears streamed unchecked down his face. I could hardly bear his grief. It is a pitiful thing to see a big man break down and sob.

Later that evening, Paul and I were finally able to talk about Melissa and her problem. We haltingly began to clothe with words our acceptance of the present and our fears for the future—a calm after the emotional storm. Our ignorance was appalling. We knew nothing about the world of the handicapped. But there was no denial of the truth. We held out no hope that the diagnosis was faulty.

We talked about the doctor's suggestion of placing Melissa in an institution. But the mere thought of handing over our particular burden to strangers ran against the grain of our hearts. We thought we should take our imperfect angel home.

It was difficult to separate our emotions from rational thought. There were no guidelines for us to follow. And, quite clearly, we knew that the problem was too big for us. We were up against a blank wall. And so we prayed. It was all we knew to do.

*God, Melissa is yours. You sent her; we don't know why, but the way is pretty dark. You must have your reasons.*

The pivotal question seemed to be whether or not we should take Melissa home or find a home or school that would train her properly. We considered our four children at home and the solemn responsibility we had to them. We thought about the recent emotional trauma each had experienced in the death of their baby sister Martha almost three years ago.

How would living with a retarded sister affect their lives? Would we end up devoting too much time and attention to this small baby at their expense? They were at a most vulnerable stage of maturation. I could so easily envision them bringing their friends home and I wondered if they would be ashamed of Melissa. Would they be embarrassed? Would they feel that they, too, might someday have a baby that was handicapped?

Then the pendulum would swing back again. The feeling of guilt that accompanied the thought of giving our baby up was overwhelming. Would we be side-stepping our parental duties? And what about the fear of outside censure?

What would our friends and neighbors think? Would they be critical? It would be much easier to win their respect and admiration if we brought Melissa home, gave up our outside activities, and dedicated ourselves to the care of this special child with her unique needs.

We realized that our feelings of guilt should not dictate our choice. Melissa would always need someone to care for her physical and educational needs. She was entitled to the privilege of associating with people on her own level, with similar mental and social capabilities.

Had we a right to isolate her in a cocoon, albeit a cocoon of love? And what about the chilling fact that we might not always be here to look after her? I was forty-two and Paul was forty-three. We had to plan realistically for her future.

Pearl Buck, in *The Child Who Never Grew*, says it all so simply: "The world is not shaped for the helpless."

Finally we came to the most important truth of all: Keeping Melissa at home with us would not make her any more "accepted," nor would placing her in a special home make her any more "rejected."

So it was that, later that night, long past visiting hours, we solemnly decided to place Melissa in a home for retarded children. And we wept even as we said the words so quietly to one another.

At five-thirty the following morning, as the wheels of the baby carts were squeaking happily down the corridors, I made a quick decision. When the nurse brought baby Melissa to me to nurse, I said I had decided not to breastfeed, asking instead for a bottle of formula. But I was consumed with grief as she lay so helplessly by my side, trying to suck on the over-sized nipple of her bottle. I felt I was betraying my own flesh and blood. Each meal grew progressively worse. I could no longer find the small opening to her mouth, my eyes awash with tears and my breasts aching to be emptied.

The following morning I asked if they would please feed her in the nursery. Still, I could not keep myself away. Tottering down the hall to the nursery, I stood leaning against the large picture window and watched a young nurse cuddle my baby in her arms. And it hurt, because I should have been the one holding Melissa.

*What is happening to me? What am I doing to myself? Am I rejecting her? Or am I trying not to tangle up my heart with the weight of our decision?*

I felt I could not discover any inner reservoir of strength if I did not stoically prepare myself, even now, for the coming days of separation.

*Oh God, you have placed in my arms a strange burden. I can't fully see the size or the shape of it, but I know that you have tailored it to fit. You made my frame and you must have remembered that I am not very strong. Help me not to forget what I have known about you for so long a time. Please help!*

An uncontrollable trembling seized me. I willed myself to be still—so still that I could hear the throbbing of my heart against my eardrums. I listened, straining. There was no voice from on high, no whisper in the winds, just a very matter-of-fact nurse's voice coming from somewhere behind me.

"Come, you had better go back to your room now."

# 2

I lay back on the hospital bed and closed my eyes, thinking about our family and about a very painful moment three years ago that tested our faith.

It was on a Monday morning that it happened, the sixteenth of May. The date was important, because it also happened to be my mother's birthday. Dear Mother was living so far away that, as yet, she had not even seen our latest baby, six-month-old Martha. But she and Father were driving up from Florida the first week in June, to see this late-in-life wonder, our fifth child.

It was a made-to-order Monday. A bright sun and brisk breezes flapped the diapers on the clothes line. I laid Martha down for a morning nap in her carriage. Kissing the moist, fat crease at the back of her neck, I watched her gratefully stretch her baby body out flat as I tucked the blanket around her well-padded bottom. Tugging the mosquito netting around the hood of the carriage, I looked at my watch: eleven o'clock.

I flew indoors to attack my housework with renewed vigor. Spring fever! When the beds were made and dishes popped into the dishwasher, I loaded the coffeemaker. Into the oven went coffeecake. I could hardly wait to see my two friends who were driving down from North Jersey. Even before I had time to find my favorite mugs, I heard the sound of tires crushing the pebbles in the driveway. They must have made excellent time on the New Jersey Turnpike.

We sat at the kitchen table, drinking coffee and nibbling the coffeecake, our conversation nonstop. I babbled about all the new things Martha was doing, and they listened attentively, as though this were the first time these feats had been performed.

15

They didn't act bored, so I blithely occupied center stage. Suddenly I jumped to my feet.

"It's twelve, do you believe it? Time for Martha's bottle. I'll go and bring her in."

They smiled expectantly. I looked through the screen door of the kitchen. The carriage was just a few feet away, the netting billowing gently in the wind. At the birdfeeder, a tufted titmouse cracked open a sunflower seed. The sun was almost overhead and it warmed my bare arms. It was the last time I felt warm that day.

Kneeling on the ground, I peeked in through the slit of the hood. We so often played peek-a-boo, but this time, it was different. There was no response. Martha did not lift her head. She simply lay there face down in her carriage.

I tore at the netting frantically and turned her over. Her tiny face was puffy. Her closed eyes were bluish-colored and swollen. I grabbed her from the depths of her carriage. Her head flopped backwards, and she lay limp and lifeless in my arms like a rag doll.

I screamed. At the top of my lungs, I let out an eerie, disbelieving wail that must have rent the heavens in two.

*Did you hear my cry, God? Was that a clap of thunder? Or just the sound of my heart breaking in a million pieces?*

I simply could not believe that this thing, this awful thing was happening to me, to my baby. I stumbled into the kitchen with my bundle of death and placed her wordlessly into the arms of my friend, Marge. Frantically, she loosened Martha's clothing and laid her on the kitchen table. With her mouth over Martha's mouth, Marge poured her breath into my baby's lungs. It was of little use; there was no response.

My thoughts flew to my husband, my Paul. I had to tell Paul. I dialed his number. His place of business was twenty miles away. I prayed that he would not have left for lunch.

I heard his voice on the other end of the line, and broke into tears. My words were garbled, but the message was all too clear.

*Something has happened to our precious baby, our new love.*

Paul drove home breaking all speed limits. Somehow, he kept believing that, when he got there, everything would be all right. But it never would be all right, ever again.

What followed was a nightmare. The ambulance sirened its arrival, and the steady hissing of the respirator joined the other confusing noises in our kitchen: the hushed whispering of neighbors, the matter-of-fact pronouncements of the paramedic, the steady ringing of the phone.

But little Martha lay there, so still. People surrounded her naked smallness with pity, trying so hard to coax her back to living again. They wouldn't give up, and that was an added hell for me. We stood watching, not touching. An eternity slipped by.

And then they simply turned off the life-giving machine. It was all over. Paul and I clung to each other. There was no need for words. We were shut away from the world, encased in a little box of grief.

We walked slowly to our bedroom and shut the door. Falling to our knees by the bed, we sobbed out our grief to our heavenly Father. Our broken hearts asked the timeless question: Why? There seemed to be no rhyme or reason. There were sickly babies, unwanted or imperfect, in the world; why didn't God take one of them? But the heavens were made of lead.

The doctor spoke up, trying so hard to be calm and detached: "There will have to be an autopsy, you know. It's mandatory in New Jersey for all accidental deaths of babies under one year of age."

An autopsy? I could not grapple with the idea. It seemed macabre to search a tiny body for this, this happening, God's mistake on a sunny Monday morning in the month of May. And yet, I wanted to know. I thought about Sudden Infant Death Syndrome (SIDS), that unexplainable silent robber of small babies. Was that the reason? Or did she smother right before my very eyes?

*But Martha was healthy, she could sit up all by herself, she was learning to creep.*

"Don't you realize that the very same thing could have happened even while you were holding her? Why, yesterday in the papers, there was a case in which a ten-month-old baby died exactly . . ." the doctor's voice droned on. But my ears were deaf. There was cold comfort in the knowledge of other similar cases.

*If only I had gone out earlier! If only I had put her in her crib! If only I hadn't had company! I will never forgive myself for letting this happen.*

At the doorway, the doctor stopped and asked, "Do you have anything that you can take tonight? Sleeping pills, or a tranquilizer?"

*We used to have one, a fifteen-pound one wrapped in a pink plaid blanket. She was all we ever needed.*

I turned away and hid my face on Paul's shoulder. Then one by one, everyone left, each on his own private mission of mercy. Some went to pick up our four children at their various schools, some to whip up a hot casserole to send to us for dinner, and some to go home to pray.

And someone called a mortician. He was our next visitor, coming in by the front door and leaving by the kitchen door with his small, plaid-wrapped bundle. He said he would telephone us later. I felt a cold numbness seize my soul.

David, Bob, Diane, and Steve came running in the back kitchen door. Trying to piece together exactly what had happened, they stumbled all over themselves looking for some answers. There was nothing to say that made any sense to them.

"Why would God do that? She wasn't sick or anything."

"How did it happen?"

"Mom, where were you?"

"Did you know right away?"

Here were questions for which there were no answers. I stood there speechless; then Paul opened his arms and gathered us all to him in a cluster of misery.

It is a strange thing with grief. Precisely when you would drown yourself in it and let the waves of sorrow wash over your soul, your sorrow is broken into—by daily persistent things, like hunger or thirst, or simply by cold, bold questions that demand reasonable answers. Where is our family burial plot? Do we want a memorial service? Have we called all our relatives?

Later that afternoon, the pastor from our home church in Hawthorne, New Jersey, arrived at our front door. Quite unbidden, he proved to be an angel in disguise. With tears in his eyes, he sensed our bewilderment.

"What can I do to help?"

Since we did not have the answer even to that simple question, he asked if we had a family plot. Then he offered us a place in his own family plot: a memorial-type garden cemetery, no tombstones, a simple bronze plaque in the ground.

We were dumbfounded. We weren't even sure whether we should have a funeral service. We had never been to one. Was it the proper thing to do? One by one, our pastor answered our questions. And we were humbled by his godly wisdom.

Later that evening, unable to sleep, we decided aspirin might help. But in searching the medicine closets, we unearthed not even one lone grain.

"Let's pray," Paul suggested. Holding hands, we knelt again at the edge of the bed and asked God to give us a night of sleep. God answered that prayer and the anesthesia of sleep came to erase, however briefly, the torment of the day.

We awoke, and she was still gone. We lay there in our big bed listening, but there was no sound from the nursery. The house was so quiet, it literally swallowed us up. I stumbled from the bed and went over to the bureau.

There was a pink diaper pin on top of my comb. I pushed it aside and combed my hair. The face that looked back at me from the mirror was drawn and haggard, the eyes were cold and despairing. I was not needed; my baby was gone.

Steve tiptoed in and stood in the doorway watching me. Then he ran to me and threw his arms around me. I felt his fierce young strength and wondered if he could sense my weakness.

"Steve, she left such a big hole in our family. What will we ever do?"

"God will fill that hole, Mom, you wait and see," he said triumphantly, with all the wisdom of his ten years.

While dressing that evening to go to the funeral home, I missed Paul. I called his name, but it stuck in my throat. Peering into the darkened nursery, I saw Paul standing by the crib, his big shoulders hunched over a pink plaid blanket bundled up in his arms. He was rocking it back and forth, singing softly under his breath with tears streaming down his face.

"Oh Paul, please don't do that to yourself."

Almost automatically, he folded the blanket and placed it neatly at one end of the empty crib.

All too soon, the day of the funeral came. And it was a miserable day, raining on and off, as if the heavens just couldn't stop crying.

We drove to the funeral home, an old-fashioned square house with a wraparound porch. We didn't expect many people to be there, for we had just moved to the area two months ago. But there were our neighbors whom we scarcely knew and some dear friends from North Jersey.

I walked hand-in-hand with Paul up to the casket. There was Martha, and yet she wasn't there. All that was left was the small body that she had lived in, oh so briefly.

Such a beautiful home God had loaned her to live in: the clear baby skin, the round cheeks, the fine new hair, the chubby legs and pudgy arms. I reached out and touched the tiny pink ribbon in her hair. Her pink ruffled dress stood away from her body as if someone had just starched and ironed it. I touched her bare arm; it was cold and hard. This was the feeling of death.

Diane tucked a small pink rose in one hand. "To take to Jesus," she whispered in Martha's tiny ear.

I had this awful feeling that if I took my eyes away from her, she would roll over and dash to pieces on the floor. She was not dead, only sleeping in this strange place. Perhaps I was having some kind of terrible nightmare, and, in a moment, if I could hang on, I would wake up and find her back in my arms again.

Our minister began to read from the Bible.

Suffer the little children, and forbid them not, to come unto me, for of such is the kingdom of heaven.

Except ye be converted and become as little children, ye shall not enter into the kingdom of heaven.

My soul stood on tiptoe to listen. I drank in his words like a thirsty sponge. And then, like the old Scottish woman who would throw her apron over her head to "be alone in her tabernacle with her God," I wanted nothing more than aloneness. I needed to talk with my God.

*Baby Martha has finished her life's work. She doesn't have to try to "become as little children" . . . she is one, a tiny little lamb that has gone home to her heavenly Father.*

A hush swept over my soul. I wanted to fall down and worship my God. Clenching both my thumbs tightly, I shot up an intense little plea for understanding and forgiveness.

*It's OK, God, I don't need to know why you did it.*

Then came that awesome moment when they tucked the white satin quilt around her small body and slowly, oh so slowly, closed the lid of the casket. A hushed period to the sentence of death.

It was a seventy-mile ride to the cemetery. We rode together in our family car. David, Bob, Diane, and Steve sat looking out the rain-streaked windows as the wet roads passed by. There was no talking. I think they did not know exactly the right thing to say, and, feeling that any words spoken on this eventful day should be right words, there was silence.

We could have been any ordinary family out for a Sunday afternoon ride—only our littlest one rode on ahead of us in a black hearse.

Diane pressed her tear-stained face against the window. "Just think," she cried, "I have a sister up in heaven."

Nobody spoke.

"Remember what we used to do when Martha had her diphtheria shots and wouldn't stop crying?"

Diane kept right on: "We'd sing to her, remember?"

The agony needed to be lessened, so we sang each of her favorite songs: the special ones that we waltzed her around the living room to and the Sunday school ones that we all knew so well.

> Jesus loves me, this I know . . .
> Jesus wants me for a sunbeam . . .
> Jesus loves the little children . . .

We walked over the sodden grass to huddle under the green canopy. As we laid the tiniest member of our family in the ground, we knew we were depositing our first treasure up in heaven.

For where your treasure is,
There will your heart be also.

# 3

The soul has a desolate desert. I discovered mine after the hurricane of emotion had stopped churning. In its wake was a calm so tenacious that I could deal dry-eyed and grim-lipped with the half-filled can of Johnson's baby powder, the white shoes never worn, the too-new crib unmarked by tiny teeth. A calm so frail that it could be shattered by the merest scrap of a lullaby or a baby's sob.

I scarcely had time to pack away her baby world when I received a call from John, the pastor of the church we were attending.

His words were hesitant. "Mildred, I know you have hardly had time to recover from Martha's home-going, but something happened today which I simply must share with you. A young lady, married to an overseas soldier, gave birth to a baby girl just three weeks ago. The baby is born out of wedlock, so she does not want her husband to know."

I could tell by his barely concealed enthusiasm that his words were a doorway to something much more exciting. But I said nothing.

"She and her mother brought the baby over to us, and left her. The baby is downstairs right now, in our living room. The mother wants to place the baby in a Christian home for adoption."

I started to cry softly.

"I know your grief is fresh, but I couldn't help thinking of you folks, and wondering . . ." his voice trailed off.

"Did you say she was just three weeks?" I asked, swallowing hard. "What color eyes does she have? Does she have any hair yet?"

At the end of my babbling, I stopped dead. "But how will I

know, pastor, if this is what God really wants for us?"

John spoke slowly. "We will pray with you. Today is Friday. She would like an answer by Sunday."

*Is this the way you work, God? Would you take away my baby and give me somebody else's baby to bring up?*

I reassured John that we too would indeed pray about this momentous decision, as I placed the receiver quietly back on the wall. I resolved not to tell the kids. I knew for certain what their reaction would be.

But that afternoon, the minute they popped in the back door, my willpower vanished. They stood open-mouthed, as I shared with them the phone call from our pastor.

"Can you believe God?" from David.

"That is the most incredible news!" This was Bob.

"How soon can we go and get her?" Steve and Diane, as with one voice.

I tried to slow them down, explaining that we didn't know yet if this was God's will for our lives.

"Oh Mom, come on, we've never had a brand-new baby given to us before. How could you even think this is not God's will for us?"

"Mom, the baby is just three weeks old!"

"I know, I know," I mumbled.

"I don't believe you, Mom, how could it *not* be God's will?"

"And—and—how will you ever know? This baby has just got to be for us." It was a symphony of protest.

I admitted it would not be easy, but I knew that God would give peace in my heart if this was what he wanted for our family.

When I told Paul that night over dinner, he was equally as enthusiastic as the rest of the family—and just as certain that we could not arrive at any objective decision in the light of our mercurial emotions. We needed to pray and then wait for God to show us.

Saturday, I went food shopping. But my mind was not on meat and potatoes for our Sunday dinner. My eyes were searching for babies, perched in many of the shopping carts. Each time I spotted one, I gazed longingly at an innocent face

24

and yearned to scoop each baby up and shower it with hugs and kisses, just to take my aching away.

*How will it feel? Will she fit into our family? Can she fill that empty niche?*

The thought of having a baby again in our home sent my spirits soaring. I almost felt pregnant!

Saturday night, there was another telephone call, this time from Janet, our pastor's wife.

"I am truly embarrassed at having to ask this favor of you, but guess what, I need a babysitter. I have to teach my Sunday-school class of twelve girls tomorrow morning."

There was a brief moment of hesitation.

"And I got to thinking that maybe this might be an ideal opportunity for you to be alone with the baby and see how you feel about adopting her. What do you think? Will it be too hard for you?"

I gulped. "No . . . yes . . . why, sure, I'll help you out. What time do you want me there?"

That Sunday morning, I walked into the parsonage and was handed a bottle of formula. The pastor's wife took me upstairs to the bedroom where a little dark-haired baby girl was nestled between two pillows atop a big double bed.

Janet left and I was alone with this precious little unwanted angel. I leaned over the bed and watched her stretch her legs as she slept somewhat fitfully. Looking her over carefully, I could see that she was a beautiful baby. Three weeks old, I mused. It had been exactly three weeks ago that our Martha had died.

Could this possibly be just a coincidence, or was it something so carefully orchestrated that we would not miss God's perfect plan for our lives? I sang a little Swedish lullaby and patted her as she snuggled against my left shoulder. She gave a resounding burp.

But even as she nuzzled in my neck, I knew this was somebody else's baby. Could I ever love her as my own? Or would I just try to make believe that she was my own Martha? Was I being presumptuous? Or one step ahead of God? I knew God was not in the habit of giving back what he chose to take away. I felt no surge of longing sweep over me, no desire to clutch her to me and never let her go. I only knew that somehow, some strange and awe-filled way, this baby was not meant for me. There was nothing but tumult inside.

But how could I ever tell my family? I despised people who made decisions based on feelings alone. Their reasoning sounded so smug and complacent. Nobody could argue with inner feelings—who would dare tear down that fortress? It seemed an unfair way of winning a battle, especially when making the incontestable declaration: "It's not God's will for my life." Who among us could dare argue against that?

On the way home from church, I calmly announced to the family that I did not feel that adopting this baby was the right thing for us to do.

Their mouths hung open in disbelief. Questions flew at me from all corners of our car.

"I don't believe you, Mom. Here God sends you a replacement baby—well almost—and you say you don't think it's his will, that it's not meant to be. How do you know? Why are you so sure?"

And even as I explained, I knew that to them I must sound woefully unconvincing.

"All I can say," I replied, somewhat lamely, "is that I know God promises inner peace. No, I don't expect God to write his answer in the skies. But I just have this inner gnawing conviction that it simply isn't right for us."

They digested my explanation in silence. The rest of the day was a wash-out. I felt ostracized from my own family. I knew Diane, perhaps more than the rest, was deeply disappointed. She wanted a sister so much.

Monday rolled around, and my own spirits hit the downward trail. Doubts and misgivings occupied center stage.

Tuesday. Not much better.

Wednesday. The telephone rang about eleven that morning. It was Janet.

"You'll never guess what happened this morning, just about an hour ago. I can't believe it, Mildred. I'm so glad you didn't take that baby home."

"Why? What happened to her?" My heart was in my throat.

"Oh, the baby is just fine; she slept like a little angel last night. But around ten this morning, her mother, grandmother, and lawyer all appeared on my front doorstep. They had come to take the baby home."

"Home?" I repeated inanely.

"Yes, her mother had changed her mind about allowing her baby to be adopted. She has decided to tell her husband everything."

I tried to envision the scene that had taken place at the parsonage. I was speechless. Janet kept talking.

"So that dear little baby just this moment departed! Are you terribly disappointed?" Janet's tone was most solicitous. I think she was expecting me to cry.

All I could say was, "Janet, I can hardly believe what you are saying. God is so good to me. He knew I didn't need another heartache just now. That's why he never even let me take her home. I can't imagine what it would have been like, falling in love again, and then having another baby snatched out of my arms."

"Oh Janet, thank you, thank you!" I babbled incoherently. I hung up the phone. Waves of relief flooded my soul.

*Thank you, God. You didn't let me down!*

# 4

All that was almost three years ago. Lying in the hospital, alone with my brand-new sorrow, I was swept away by waves of sadness.

*Another heartache, a fresh one to replace the old—Melissa!*

A few days later, I was discharged from the hospital. The sunshine was everywhere that morning as we said our shaky goodbyes. My husband carried my suitcase and I held a potted yellow chrysanthemum in my hands.

Down at the end of the long hospital corridor our five-day-old baby was sleeping peacefully in the nursery. I could not bring myself to bid her goodbye.

*What horrendous deed am I about to perform? What unnatural love is spilling out from my mother-heart to enable me to leave my handicapped baby for strangers to care for? How can I walk out of this hospital empty-armed? I've paid my dues: nine months of pregnancy, eight hours of excruciating labor. I have a right to something or someone. But my arms are empty.*

Our children had been devastated by our decision.

Our oldest boy, David, a junior in a New York college, had been visiting at the home of his fiancee, Kathy, in a small town near Montreal, when Paul reached him by phone to tell him the distressing news about Melissa. David was stunned. When he hung up the receiver he blurted out the news to Kathy's family.

"Our new baby, Melissa, is . . . retarded!"

David retreated into a tower of silence. He was not even sure exactly what a baby with Down syndrome looked like. He told us later that his mind was permeated with visions of a baby with a large head, distorted features, and slanted eyes.

When dinner was at last over, David quickly grabbed Kathy's doctor-father by the arm and together they walked downstairs to his private office.

"Does this mean that Kathy and I might have a retarded baby, too?"

Gently Kathy's father explained the happenstance of this chromosomal abnormality. "Melissa has received the damning gift of one extra chromosome at the time of conception. Her blood cells will continue to divide and reproduce in the same imperfect manner, thus establishing as an irrevocable trust, her sad inheritance. Your mother, David, ran an extra risk of having a baby with Down syndrome because of her age. Her chances were one in fifty."

"Did she know this?"

"That is a question you will have to ask your mother yourself."

David's fears were somewhat quieted, but later that evening he broke down and sobbed in Kathy's arms.

Each of our children, in his or her own way, accepted the double-barreled blast of grief, remembering the loss of baby Martha, and questioning the why of baby Melissa. We were grateful that they did not challenge our decision to place Melissa in a private home for the mentally handicapped.

We did not talk with them about her prognosis simply because we did not know the answers to their questions. It was a whole new world for all of us. We would have to discover it together. And strangely enough, in 1964 there was not a wealth of information that was readily available.

Precious little comfort was to be found in the sympathy of our friends. I really think that their lack of knowledge equaled ours. Many of them could easily be put into the category of the prophet Job's "miserable comforters."

A woman phoned me while I was still in the hospital and offered what she considered to be comforting words: "Well, if you had to have a retarded baby, thank God she's a mongoloid. When she grows up, she will love to do housework. I knew one once who would wash the walls over and over. . . ."

I shut my ears. I was not looking for a housekeeper.

"They're the best of all of them, believe me, they're funny and lovable—kind of like little clowns. It'll work out: you wait and see."

There was no acknowledgment of our sorrow or even a passing comment about our decision to place Melissa in a home. We were clearly out on a limb, all by ourselves.

One dear friend stands out for his rare insight. Joe Bayly had visited me in the hospital. He just stood there in the doorway of my room and said two words: "I'm bruised!"

Joe had suffered. He knew what it was to be struck not once, not twice, but three times by calamities beyond the scope of his imagination. Joe was hurting because I was hurting. And that was really all I wanted: understanding love. I needed just an arm around my shoulder or a quick hug, not someone to preach to me, or philosophize.

Our decision to place Melissa in a home would now have to be accompanied by action. Where was this place that would qualify as our baby Melissa's other home? Where were the people who would gather her in their arms and train her and love her in the way that we would have?

Paul took three days off from work the following week and he and I started out early each morning on our mission. Our goal was to visit as many private and state mental health facilities in our area as possible. It was no easy task.

I will not soon forget the day that we visited our first state-run institution in Pennsylvania. Here, we were told, almost three thousand retarded of all ages lived. And there was a waiting list of nearly seven thousand. This thought alone staggered our minds.

Acres of green lawns and wooded areas surrounded the complex of rectangular brick buildings. A network of macadam roads threaded their way around the tired-looking structures.

We kept looking for small children, and when I spotted a group of what appeared to be fifty or more boys, playing in an open field, I asked Paul to pull over. We got out of the car and walked to the edge of the playground.

"What are they doing?" I frowned.

They seemed to be milling about uncertainly, dressed in an odd assortment of what appeared to be castoff clothing. Some older men were wearing ladies' dresses that flapped around their ankles.

Seated on a bench under a large spreading maple sat a gray-haired woman in a white uniform. From time to time she raised her head to exhale a long puff of smoke. She did not see us or anyone else, for that matter.

One small cluster of men was engaged in an activity of their own making. A young boy and older man were the main contestants. They lay together on the ground, locked in a frenzied embrace. Their movements were rhythmical. The rest of the group circled around them and were content to watch and call out words and names that I could not make out. It was probably just as well.

I watched with a kind of fascination while slowly it began to dawn on me what was happening. I shuddered. Paul put his arm around me and gently led me back to the car. Neither one of us spoke.

We were not permitted to tour inside the buildings without a guide. A young girl was assigned to this responsibility and we followed in her wake like two mechanized dolls.

"Would you like to see the crib area?"

"Oh yes," I said eagerly.

The sand and grit under our heels on the concrete steps and halls made a scraping sound. Through an oversized metal door we entered a dormitory with row upon row of chipped, painted cribs. I guess I expected to see small babies or even toddlers. But in each crib was a body with arms and legs and a face with eyes—shipwrecks of humanity of assorted ages huddled in smelly, sodden diapers and tattered gray undershirts. Some were just as they came into this world: stark naked.

It was like entering another world, a world where bodies grew and minds stood still, a world where troubled minds could not control twisting bodies, where eyes could not focus, and where heads grew too large or forever remained too small.

It was a grotesque world, with people who banged their heads against their barred prisons, slapped their own bodies, or simply screamed. Nobody seemed to pay attention, so they screamed all the louder. And in my heart, I screamed, too, at my God.

*Are these part of your creation, God? What happened? What have you done? Where have you been?*

Our guide unlocked the doors to the dayroom, a large

cement-floored room with benches around the edges. Long tables were scattered here and there, but there were no chairs in sight to sit on. This, I was told, was their playroom. But I could see no toys or playthings.

"What do they do all day?"

Nobody heard the question. The moment we entered the room, we were swallowed up by the clamoring children. I could not understand what they were saying as they reached out to grab us. I wanted to pull away or unclasp their fingers, but somehow I did not dare, for it would be like rejecting my own Melissa.

"Which ones have Down syndrome?" I asked.

She pointed them out, calling them the "best of the lot."

But her words were small comfort.

After that breakthrough into the world of "perpetual children," we started to visit private facilities. We still did not know exactly what to expect, but we discovered waiting lists everywhere, crowded conditions, high monthly costs, and a seeming lack of honest-to-goodness love or concern. A macabre world of dreary routine, bed making, diaper changing, and meal feeding, it left us chilled to the bone.

Then, quite unexpectedly, we heard of a children's home in the midwest. Friends of ours in Ohio spoke of it with the highest of praise. It was run by the Mennonite Church. On the basis of their glowing recommendation, we made application for Melissa to be admitted.

Their policies, however, dictated that she be admitted directly to this home upon hospital discharge. That meant we could not have her in our home for even a small while.

This seemed, to us, a very unusual requirement.

# 5

The dreaded morning dawned. The sun rose, a tired breeze blew now and again. This was the morning that our twenty-three-day-old Melissa was to leave the sterile world of the hospital and enter her own special sphere of the handicapped.

It was that terrible, dreadful morning when our sad family gathered in our driveway around the car to see our small baby for the very first time, to bid her goodbye almost before saying hello.

They came, wearing robes over their pajamas, in bare feet and with sleep-creased faces. They huddled in silent homage around the white wicker basket wedged on the back seat of the car. They viewed her through the magnifying lenses of their own emotions, gently pulling back her soft pink blanket to touch her small bare feet or pink arms.

Steve maneuvered his big thumb inside the clasp of her fist and stood mutely, his dark brown eyes flooding with tears.

*How can it be that this small one, our baby, so innocent, so seemingly perfect, how can it be that she is retarded?*

Watching the tears flow unchecked down my mother's cheeks, I knew that she did not understand the wisdom of the impending separation. I could almost feel her grandmother's heart reaching out to enfold this child with the broken wing. And my father stood there, somewhat apart, bewildered and reluctant to face the full impact of our decision.

"It's time now. We must get started."

It was Paul, bringing down the final curtain on this desolate scene. Our farewells were automatic. We departed without further fanfare. There is just so much grief that a family can stand.

It was a ten-hour trip by automobile, but Melissa never once cried. I cuddled her almost fiercely. My tears splashed down on her upturned face, and she blinked in wonder. I examined her face over and over, but each feature seemed perfect. Inside I felt tied in knots of agony.

I did not know that I had the capacity to weep for such a long period. By the end of our journey, I was physically and emotionally exhausted.

When we reached the small town and spotted the home set back from the road in a cluster of trees, I panicked.

"Please drive by," I begged Paul. "I just can't do it. It's wrong—totally, terribly wrong!"

He parked the car at the edge of the road and together we held our small baby and wept. How long we sat there, I do not know. There were no audible words of prayer. But we knew that God was with us in that car.

Melissa grew restless in our arms and Paul reached over and switched on the ignition. We drove back again to the square white house, very slowly.

There were three short steps in the front. We walked up numbly, like robots. Before our hands had touched the door-knob, a round-faced nurse met us at the front door with a big smile.

"Well, if it isn't our new baby all the way from Pennsylvania. May I hold her? My, if she isn't the cutest little pumpkin. Mary, come here and see this adorable . . ."

And so it went. It was like showing off any baby to adoring relatives.

Before we knew it, we were in a nursery with three picture windows and twenty-two stainless steel cribs. The babies ranged from one month to three years. Here were babies suffering birth defects and brain damage, as well as cerebral palsy.

"Strange company to leave you with, my small one," I whispered over and over, "but Melissa, this is your world, different from ours but very, very special. You belong here, my love. Here you will have friends just like you."

The corner of a yellow patchwork quilt was turned back on Melissa's crib. We gratefully watched her stretch. Then we inspected the rest of the home.

Fourteen children with Down syndrome, about ten or twelve years old, were seated in yet another room around a low table, feeding themselves, sloppily but happily. Each one had a big towel bib running from under his chin to his plate. It was much like any family dinner table. Everybody was jabbering at once. Later, these same children in bathrobes and pajamas sat on the floor in front of a television set. Everywhere there were signs of love and care.

It was everything our friends had reported. Our hearts were content. Here was a place where we could be sure that Melissa would be safe and happy.

But that did not make it any easier to leave her there the next day. When I bent over her crib to kiss her soft cheek, she was sleeping soundly. I looked at her for a long moment. As I turned and walked away, I felt I was ripping out my own heart.

Our return five-hundred-mile trip was bleak. Neither of us felt much like speaking.

Thumping our suitcases on the kitchen floor, the first thing my eyes lit upon was our calendar. It was one of those calendars that has each day printed on a separate page, to tear off when that day has passed. In bold black letters, it spelled out the month *September* and the day *Tuesday* and the numeral *three.*

I drew in my breath sharply. Time had stopped on the day of Melissa's birth. Under the date there was a Bible verse, "I shall yet praise him." I ripped it off and threw it into the waste basket.

*Praise God for a mentally-handicapped child? No, there will be no praise for Melissa from me, God.*

The next morning, the doorbell chimed and a special delivery letter from Texas was handed to us.

Words written on a piece of paper and sent twelve-hundred miles away somehow don't seem very adequate. We certainly have been praying for you as you search for a home for Melissa. We put our heads together and decided that maybe we could do something concrete and useful by urging you to come and spend a few days with us in Big D. So we are enclosing two pieces of paper that might help. They are strictly first class (don't drink the liquor) and family plan (which means you can't travel on Sunday) and on a jet direct from you to us. The rest is up to you. Fill in the date and let us know. If you could come soon, you might relax around the pool. And if I could think of any more enticements, I'd include them, too. But then, I'm a theologian, not a sales manager.

It seemed that they were the most beautiful words we had ever read. Charles was one of those prized possessions: a dear friend. He was indeed a theologian, a doctor of philosophy, and author of many books.

It did not take us long to fill in the missing dates. Soon we were enjoying a complete switch of environment and change of pace. The therapy of sharing openly our doubts and misgivings over the momentous decision we had made hastened the healing process.

Six days later, back in Pennsylvania, we felt whole and strong again. Life was the same curious mixture of the mundane and the momentous that it always had been.

Shopping trips to supermarkets suddenly turned out to be another hurdle in my acceptance process. On my very first trip, I noticed a tiny baby asleep on the cold wire bottom of a shopping cart. Cans and boxes of breakfast cereal were piled helter-skelter around him. An older brother, grabbing whatever he could reach on the shelves, dropped his booty into the basket.

I stood there looking for their mother and found a young girl, her head outlined in pink curlers, standing nearby, pinching heads of lettuce at the vegetable counter. Now and again she angrily scolded the baby's mischievous brother.

I seethed. It took all the strength I could muster not to snatch the baby out of the cart, or scold the mother about caring so little for her precious child. Surely her little one would be dashed and dented long before her shopping was complete.

Tears stung my eyes as I left my half-filled cart in the aisle and bolted out of the store, hardly remembering what I had come for.

Our house was so empty. Babies leave an enormous void in a family.

Endless ages passed before we could drive out to Ohio to see our baby. And even a visit to Melissa proved to be shattering. The ten hours it took us to drive the many miles to Ohio were fatiguing. And by the end of the trip we could hardly wait to see and hold our baby.

Many times we arrived well past visiting hours, but they had assured us that we were welcome "any time." We took them at their word.

One evening we arrived in Ohio around ten in the evening, bone weary. The lights were dimmed. We tiptoed through the quiet halls past the sleeping sounds of the children. Paul, with his long strides, was always a step ahead of me.

When we got to the nursery, I walked over to the crib by the picture window where we had left her when we first came.

"Paul, is this . . . our Melissa?" I pawed through my purse to find my glasses.

"Honey, no!" His voice was gentle. "That isn't our baby! They must have moved her crib. Here she is fast asleep right by the door, see?"

I walked away from the small stranger that I had been looking at with a sigh of relief. But my heart gave a sickening lurch as I picked up our own Melissa and held her fiercely. She had changed so much.

Melissa's face was a curious mix of young and old. Her eyes did not focus on ours for long. Her body was warm and passive so we simply held her all the more tightly as we walked and rocked her. It was all we had. We peered down into the other cribs with Melissa in our arms.

Many were misshapen in body with twisted limbs or large, ungainly heads: cribs filled with heartaches.

On our trip back home the next day, we did not talk much. Paul's face was grim as he maneuvered back and forth in the Sunday traffic. I stared through the side window listlessly.

"You know, Paul, there should be a home like that in our part of the country—a home where love is felt." The statement hung there between us and no comment was made for many miles.

Our visits came and went so swiftly. And there were always the goodbyes. The scar tissue covering our wounds was so thin that each time we had to leave, the scabs were torn off and we suffered all over again. The healing process was seemingly endless.

A few months later, during a shopping trip to buy some new clothes for our growing baby, I walked into a children's store.

"I'm looking for some little girl's overalls."

"What size do you want? We carry infant sizes from 0–3 and toddler sizes from 3–6X."

I swallowed hard.

*What size is she wearing now? I don't know; I don't know. I don't know my own baby's size.*

"Well, she's almost seven months old."

"You know, ma'am, babies vary in their rate of growth. How much does she weigh?"

My hands were wet with perspiration.

*What had they said in their last letter? I can't remember.*

"About sixteen pounds, I guess," I said in a low voice.

He gave me a long, hard look.

"Is this a gift, ma'am, or is this for your own baby?"

*My own baby? Oh yes, she is my own, yet she is five-hundred miles away and I don't know any of the little things about her that I long to know.*

I mumbled something meaningless under my breath and walked quickly out of the store.

*Why, God, do you have to send the same hurt back again and again?*

And the painful things often arrived in different disguises, so that I was never prepared ahead of time for the best way to deal with each new set of circumstances.

One evening Paul and I attended a charity dinner in a large hotel ballroom where we were seated at a table with five other couples, three of whom we had never met.

In exchanging pleasantries, the inevitable question popped up: "And how many children do you have?"

"Five," I answered.

"Terrific!" (This was back in those days when bigger was always better and a big family was the norm.)

Then the follow-up question: "And how old are they?"

"We have two in college, two in high school, and a seven-month-old baby."

"Can you believe it? Two in college and a little one on the scene again. You sure must have a new lease on life!"

I knew, if I started to explain, that I would burst into tears. But Paul jumped in the gap, and adroitly changed the subject. I did not need, or want, their passing expressions of sympathy. Yet I could not live with, what appeared to me, a denial of our retarded baby. So I have learned that direct and bare honesty is the only way to go.

Whenever family questions were asked, I would simply say, "Yes, we have five children: two in college, two in high school, and a little baby who is living in a special home in Ohio for retarded children."

I would never ever deny Melissa's existence even to a stranger. But I will admit, back in those early days, I often wondered if I were the only mother of a retarded child in all of Pennsylvania. I never saw any of these children out playing in our neighborhood in their yards, nor in church nor the market.

Surely there must be others!

*Where are they hiding?*

# 6

In the early spring our oldest boy David hitchhiked out to Ohio to see Melissa. He wrote us when he got back to college. You probably know how this trip got started. I suddenly realized that I had not seen my sister Melissa since she was twenty-three days old. So I hitchhiked all the way to Ohio. I went in to see Melissa, and I could tell right away she belonged to our family. Those big blue eyes and blond-red hair which had just been brushed. And there was a pretty ribbon stuck on top. And she smelled so good, she was a doll! I picked her up, and held her. She never cried, although I am sure she had a hard time getting used to the way her big brother held her. I fed her a bottle, and she's a good eater. When she finished, she let out a healthy burp. Then I guess she was tired of my holding her, so she hit the sack. To say the least, I have fallen in love with her. When Melissa woke up, she and I went over to see Mike in one of the other rooms. That little guy has the sweetest smile you have ever seen. Then I put Melissa on my knees and moved her legs back and forth so as to give her a muscle workout. Sunday afternoon, Melissa was all dressed up in a pair of blue pants with a little checked jumper over that. She was pretty as pink. I got some big smiles, and she seemed quite comfortable in my arms. What effect has this had upon me, personally? Well, it engendered within me a love for my sister that had previously existed only in an impersonal form. Now I know her and have held her and my love wells up within me at my own inadequacies of imparting something that I have . . . to her. My biggest problem is that I see her as a normal baby, and I keep hoping for an outside chance, that somewhere along the line someone goofed and she doesn't belong there. It is killing me. I can hardly see the keys for the tears. I can't get my mind off the hopelessness of the situation. Please do me the biggest favor in the world—write me a letter about this letter. I'm kind of upset!

Minutes later I was at the typewriter, trying to reach out long distance to heal his heartache.

I just this minute finished reading your letter about your visit to Melissa. I know how you feel, David, because we, too, have experienced those heart-tearing moments. And there is comfort in holding her warm little body close and whispering into her soft neck the never-to-be-answered question . . . why? But Dave, you can turn yourself inside out by longing for things that you cannot have.

Please don't allow yourself the luxury of thinking that maybe your little baby sister is normal. She is not normal and has no hopes of becoming normal. God does not set in motion certain laws, only to change them capriciously. But God has allowed a baby with Down syndrome to be born into our family. We don't know too much about how this will change each one of our lives.

For, even after the initial impact, the shock waves of living with the fact that we have a retarded baby will affect all of our lives. There's a long road ahead.

So often, parents and families refuse to believe the doctors or professionals and read into every action of their handicapped child: progress! "Maybe it's not as bad as they say, maybe she will grow out of it, and everything will be OK again. Doctors have been wrong before!" And they focus their whole attention on this one child, whom God has entrusted to their care, to the detriment of their normal children, as well as their spouses. Life is such a vapor, Dave. If this were all, these seventy or eighty years lived in a smutty old world filled with trouble and tears, it wouldn't be worth the strain. But, gently, God is molding us to be vessels fit for his name. I think it had to take a Melissa and a Martha for us!

We all ache to enjoy her in a normal relationship. I cannot allow my imagination this much freedom. My heart would crush to pieces all over again. But our Melissa will never know our heartache. All the pain is on our side.

And I suspect that that is a blessing in disguise! Someday her bonds will be loosed and God will make her whole again. And that will be heaven! Love, Mom.

It was that same spring that I felt compelled to resume my writing again. This time, I wanted to share the reasons why our family chose to place Melissa in a home.

Admittedly on the defensive, I decided it was high time for others to realize that there was more than one acceptable way to handle a problem of this nature. I mailed off my article to *Good Housekeeping* magazine.

I was nearly hysterical when a note of acceptance arrived with a generous check as well. The article was published in November, 1964, under the title, "The Baby Our Love Could Not Cure."

It evoked a tremendous reader response. And the editors were wonderful. They spared me the pain of handling the negative replies and forwarded the rest of the letters for me to answer personally. Challenging they were, and time consuming as well. I soon found myself corresponding with scores of broken-hearted parents all over the United States.

Many letters told of their discouraging search all over the country for suitable facilities. Here we could empathize completely. Hadn't we, too, been sickened by the smells, the puddled floors, the paint-chipped cribs? Our snug middle-aged world was beginning to expand. Already the shock wave of a Melissa was crumbling the corners of our minds. Again and again, we came around to the question, "Why shouldn't there be a place where Christ's love could be felt in our part of the country?"

Our burden grew heavier. Here was this outpouring of letters affirming what we had felt all along. Indeed, there was an undeniable lack of proper homes for the handicapped.

From this dismaying bedrock of need, there spawned a fragile dream, a dream of what we as a family could do to help solve some of these problems. We were caught up by our own enthusiastic natures, and began to start out many conversations with, "What if . . . ?" It soon blossomed into a twenty-four-hour-a-day preoccupation. We asked our friends to pray. We surely did not want to make a mistake. We knew that if God wasn't in it, it sure would be one huge blunder!

Suddenly it was December again, and Dave and Bob returned from college with their dirty laundry bags, undone term papers, and "Is that all the cookies you made?" comments as they devoured everything in sight. Christmas was coming! The holiday spirit fell on everyone.

One evening, before Paul had arrived home for dinner, we were kidding about what we most wanted for Christmas. The conversation was full of the easy banter that most grown-up families enjoy.

"I know what I want more than anything." It was Bob who spoke. His voice was very serious.

"I know, and I do, too!" they all chorused.

"Sounds to me like a conspiracy," I teased.

"No," they insisted, "it really isn't. We just want our baby sister home for Christmas."

My heart stuck in my throat, as I thought about the happy possibility. Have Melissa in our very own home? It would be too good to ever happen. And an inner voice was telling me that Paul would never hear of it. I felt sure that he would think we were weakening in our conviction that placing her in a home was the best decision for our family.

"I . . . I don't know what Dad will say."

"Well, let's all ask him—after dinner, of course!"

Paul sat there, rather stunned. Then his gray-green eyes grew misty as he said just two words: "Why not?"

Three days later, Paul and I were at the children's home in Ohio to pick up our fifteen-month-old Melissa for her Christmas vacation. I was as nervous as any new mother, packing Melissa's baby clothes for her two-week visit.

The childcare attendants I had grown to appreciate and respect for their labors of love, stood around watching us jam a goodly supply of baby items into our bulging suitcases.

"You'll never bring her back, you know," they nodded wisely.

"Oh, but we will. We believe this is the best place for her, here in her own little world. You'll see."

But they only smiled sadly, and kissed Melissa with a great tenderness. They were her mothers and now the parting was theirs. I held her all the tighter.

The ride home was so different this time. Melissa was coming home. I said it over and over, deep down, a kind of emotional chant. No matter for what period of time, I thought, this was today and we were together. Tomorrow might never come.

The family had been busy in our absence, and the third-floor bedroom next to Dave and Bob's now held what had been Martha's new crib and an emptied chest of drawers. Diane and Scubie—the blond, blue-eyed friend of Diane who had come to live with us after both of her parents had died—had added all the little girl things: stuffed animals, frilly lamps, and Martha's pink-and-white-plaid blanket with the fringes on both ends.

That evening, after the tumultuous welcome home that was accorded the new arrival, we undressed Melissa and placed her in her crib. She did not protest at her new surroundings and we tiptoed downstairs, smiling.

Later, as our household finally settled down, Paul and I were quietly doing the "cat out, dog in, lights out" routine when we heard a rhythmical pounding coming from the direction of Melissa's room.

Bounding up the stairs, we stood in her darkened room, lit only by the small night light on her dresser. Melissa was caught halfway between waking and sleeping, crouched on all fours, rocking back and forth, banging her head mechanically against the end of her crib. The room was filled with her monotone chant, a cross between a cry and a moan.

Paul moved her head away from the end of her crib and stood there soothingly humming and patting her diaper-padded bottom. Her rhythmical protests grew weaker. Melissa finally surrendered to her need for sleep and we crept out of the room. That night, we slept with our bedroom door open.

The next few days were filled with the wonder of Melissa. She was literally descended upon with all the stimulation and attention that a household of six could manage. She sat with open-mouthed astonishment at some of our antics.

But she did not laugh; neither did she smile. Her tongue protruded and we noted it with dismay. She took little interest in the toys we forced upon her, but was happiest when rocking back and forth on her haunches and sucking her thumb. Unsure of what we could do—if anything—to help her, we made an appointment with a famed neurosurgeon in our area.

"What is it that you want to hear from me?" He was direct and heartbreakingly blunt.

"That she is afflicted with Down syndrome is quite obvious. A chromosomal count is not at all necessary. She has all the facial appearances of a baby with Down syndrome."

We sat in front of his desk, Melissa bouncing on Paul's knee, and we looked at him helplessly. "Is there anything that we can do to help her?"

"Throw away her playpen, let her creep, let her discover things for herself, offer her all the stimulation you can. Treat her as your other children."

"The rocking?" I asked softly.

"Do not permit it. The motion traps her in a world of her own making and she will not relate to her surroundings. Divert her!"

And we turned to look at Melissa who had, quite without notice, thrown up on Paul's pants. I handed him her pink plaid blanket to cover it up, and we made a hasty exit.

Divert and stimulate, we did: constantly and exhaustingly. But something was beginning to happen. Melissa was coming alive. She started to creep and discover things on her own and each accomplishment was greeted with roaring approval. Melissa was leaving her valley of apathy.

Christmas was something else that year. Since our children had long ago passed the age of "see and grab" everything within reach, we had decorated our Christmas tree a bit more lavishly, with little thought of what occupied the lower branches.

Melissa discovered them all: the little treasures, the fragile baubles. Like Humpty Dumpty himself, they all came crashing down, never to be put together again. But we all were so enthralled at her progress that it seemed a small price to pay.

Before the holidays were over, she held our six hearts in her chubby baby hands. We dreaded the moment of separation. If only there were a home closer.

*Is Melissa to be our commission? Are these our marching orders?*

## 7

**B**y all accounts, it would have seemed that way. Two weeks after the Christmas holidays, when Melissa should have returned to her home in Ohio, she was still upstairs in her nursery. She had made her own little niche in our hearts that nothing could possibly fill but her own impish self.

"If we did start a home, Dad, would we only take the kids with Down syndrome, like Melissa?" That was Steve.

"And we sure don't want the old ones, right? Or the real crazy ones?"

"Diane!"

Our children were full of questions about our great new venture. Would we live in the same house with all the retarded children? Who would do all the cooking? Would Daddy stop working? Would we have enough money to pay their college tuition?

Unnamed fears were skulking in the attics of our adult minds and now they were given flesh and bones as our family verbalized what we were fearing. How would we get enough money together to buy a bigger house? And who would help us?

A few of our church friends thought that we were dabbling in social problems and intimated that perhaps we had better leave this kind of burden for the "liberal" Christians to perform. After all, didn't the liberals depend on their good works to get them into heaven?

We reminded them that the book of James in the New Testament had said it all rather well: "What use is it, my brethren, if a man says he has faith, but he has no works?"

One sweet old man asked us whether or not we were planning to evangelize the mentally retarded. And didn't we realize that these innocent children were safe under the atonement anyway? Why should we waste our time and talents in this way? Why bother? They would all be in heaven with us someday, anyway!

"You know what I wonder, Dad?" Bob was on his back on the living room floor with Melissa sprawled on his stomach, contentedly sucking her thumb.

"Why aren't there more Christian homes for retarded kids? Christians are the ones who should care more than anybody else."

"Exactly! But many Christians shy away from things that are not centered in or around the church."

"Yeah, but how come? Jesus certainly didn't act like that while he was here on earth."

"I know," Paul said reflectively, putting aside the evening newspaper. "Jesus warned us against seeing our brothers naked, cold, or hungry, saying, 'Depart in peace, be warmed and filled.' "

"Well," I offered, "maybe they avoid social problems so their lives are not a stumbling block to those who think if they are good enough, God couldn't keep them out of heaven. The Bible says: 'Man is saved by grace, through faith, and that not of yourselves, lest any man should boast.' "

"You're right, Mom!"

"But Dad, that isn't all there is to it, is it?"

"No, I think we Christians often overreact and let the pendulum swing too far in the other direction by forgetting about good works completely."

"So we need to demonstrate our faith in God by our good works."

"You got it, Bob! And remember, many of the very first hospitals and orphanages right here in America were founded by dedicated Christians—Christians who actually did put their faith to work."

"So," Bob persisted, "when we are faced with a real need, we should try to discover a way that we can help."

"True enough! I think God gave us a Melissa after the heartbreak of a Martha to stretch our own faith."

It was February when we decided to take the first big step. We set about recruiting four men to serve with us on our board of directors. Each one filled an area of expertise that we thought would be helpful to us in founding a home for retarded boys and girls.

Charles, a physician, volunteered to help us interview and screen admissions and advise us medically; "By," a lawyer, would keep us legally untangled; Ben was well qualified in the field of special education; Walter, a former president of a church-sponsored group of nursing homes, could help us out in this area.

Then came the big day: February 2, 1965. We met in our lawyer's office and went through all the business intricacies necessary for the formation of a not-for-profit, tax-exempt corporation. We decided to call it Melmark. The "Mel" was from Melissa, the "mar" from our baby Martha, and the "k" for our last name.

There it was, unwieldy on our tongues and almost embarrassing to say. It did not seem to us at times that we could ever pull it off. It sounded like a dream that would never quite materialize. Neither one of us was skilled in this field of human services. My husband had his master's degree in organic chemistry and years of experience in marketing and sales. I qualified only because I was the mother of Melissa.

These were hardly impressive credentials, by the world's standards. Well, we reasoned, we would lean hard on God and ask him for the help we needed to get our project rolling, despite our lack of confidence in our own abilities.

We held our very first board meeting on a Saturday morning, around the kitchen table in our Berwyn home. We started with coffee and coffeecake—and a lot of prayer. Soon our breakfast board meetings became an established habit.

Then we began to search for a suitable location for Melmark. We tramped in and out of homes, some tattered beauties, some forsaken shells, and some seeming to beg us silently to move in. But month after month went by and still no appropriate location had been uncovered.

As we looked at these homes, all bearing six-figure price tags, we realized we had a great need for substantial capital. To this day, I do not know why we were not dismayed at the prices. I guess it truly never occurred to us that God would not help us out with the dollars when the need materialized. In the meantime, we did what we could.

We mailed out fifty letters to those of our friends we thought would share our burden. And $7,000 trickled in. During this time of waiting and watching, we attended a fundraising dinner of the local chapter of a national advocacy group. It was a beautiful banquet, and at least a hundred or more people were in attendance.

They had a thirty-five member board. During their business meeting, they stated that their goal for next year was to raise $10,000. Various methods were suggested, one of which was to stand outside the shipyards in nearby Philadelphia with metal containers to solicit donations from the shipyard workers as they left from their shifts. I met Paul's glance and he looked at me with just a flicker of wonderment on his face.

"Are we crazy or something?" he whispered. "Do you know what we are planning to do, just the two of us?"

I nodded and smiled at him. I wasn't feeling especially confident or anything; I just didn't know how else to respond. We were trying to raise $100,000!

We had decided to sell our own splitlevel home in Berwyn and take the down payment from that to use toward the purchase of a larger home for Melmark. But we couldn't sell the home we were living in until we found a suitable location for Melmark. It was then that we became a bit discouraged.

Every realtor made no bones about our financial needs. It would take at least a $100,000 down payment to purchase any one of these mansions.

"What are we going to do, Paul?"

"Well, I think we need to approach foundations."

"We don't know anyone on their boards!"

"Well, we'll write them anyhow and try to arrange a meeting with them so that we can tell them what we are planning."

"Just a letter?"

"Yes, we'll start out that way and hope to get to meet somebody in charge."

It was a combination letter, part business and part a simple sharing of our dream of building "the home that love built" for mentally-handicapped boys and girls. We had no money of which to brag, and no philanthropists to whom we could turn.

So we prayed all the harder. I wonder sometimes if they were believing prayers; they certainly were desperate in nature. We had no other way to turn, yet we realized that, if any help were to come our way, God alone would be the one who would direct it.

We mailed out eighty letters to eighty foundations, and received forty responses—mostly negative. Three sent checks, not from their foundations, but personal checks, because they somehow were touched by our appeal. Seven of them showed a measure of interest in our project. But most responses stated that they would help us "in the future when you get established."

It was Paul who seemed most encouraged by even the slimmest of returns. A gift of $5.00, to him, showed interest on the part of the donor. And while we were waiting and praying for a suitable home for our Melmark, we added another crib to Melissa's nursery. One for Todd—a little Down syndrome baby whose mother had read my article in the *Good Housekeeping* magazine.

"We need what you're trying to do, and if there's any way I can help, I'll be more than happy." And Jan was the one who typed out all eighty letters to the foundations.

Not too long after that, another Down syndrome baby girl named Terry was entrusted to our care. God was seeing to it that we had our special family even before we found our special home.

The addition of these two babies into our family life stretched the patience of all of us. Yes, we did have the competent help of Elizabeth, who commuted daily from Philadelphia, but that was only weekdays from nine to five. All three little rascals, including our Melissa, had discovered that evenings and weekends were great times for some overdue whining or crying.

Todd had taken a particular liking to waking up early in the morning with his very different cry. There seemed to be no place left in the house away from the sounds of his insistent voice. We moved his playpen into a corner of our dining room, and transferred his noisy little self to this interesting spot, so that we all did not have to wake up the same time as he did—which was usually around five in the morning!

Soon it was December again. There had been such a lack of forward Melmark motion, so many slammed doors in our faces, that we were almost afraid to believe that God was working behind the scenes.

But the day before Christmas dawned and, quite without notice, things suddenly right-about-faced. Paul and Bob drove down to Berwyn to check our Melmark post office box. There were two letters. One contained a check for $2,000 from a foundation in Nebraska, and in the other letter was a personal check from a very wealthy lady in Delaware for $25,000.

I must have counted the zeroes a zillion times. We laughed and cried and ran through the house like banshees. Melissa took one look at us, covered up her eyes, and began to howl. Bob swooped her up in his big arms and hugged her tight. Then we all fell to our knees around the bed and prayed together. Our words were indistinct with happy tears, but I think God understood every single word. Finally we could afford a modest down payment. Our humble assets had grown to $87,000, enough to provide working capital as well as start-up costs.

Then we found it! At the end of our patience, at the end of our short-sighted faith, we visited a handsome thirty-five-room mansion on twenty acres of beautiful countryside with an outdoor swimming pool and large spacious hallways. And it was painted pink—the pink chateau! It was a copy of the Mal Maison in France, the castle that Napoleon gave to Josephine.

There was a walking garden to one side with pathways criss-crossing under linden trees. Nestled alongside this was a forlorn tennis court which had not heard "fifteen-love" for many a year. There was also a breathtaking thirty-by-fifty outdoor swimming pool. True, the cement was chipped and the surrounding patio slates were in a state of upheaval, but there it was, waiting for someone to love it enough to tidy it up and repair all the damage.

52

As we walked from room to room on Oriental rugs of every hue and design, it was apparent that the beautiful old home had gone through some dramatic changes. In the corner of the ballroom the furniture had been shoved into one corner, mattresses and bed springs made a unique playhouse, wheelchairs served as automobiles, and the forty-six-foot ballroom floor was their drag strip.

But it was tailored to fit our needs. There was an elevator, two fire escapes, emergency lighting and exit signs, handrails in the wide halls, and even a commercial stove in the kitchen. It was being operated as a retirement home for people with financial means, which meant that it already had a special zoning exception. And that, we had already discovered, was the most important asset.

Another invaluable asset, we soon found out, was the unprecedented publicity that my next article, called "Melissa Comes Home" (again published in *Good Housekeeping),* gave us. It was as though we had received the Good Housekeeping Seal of Approval (which we later did receive). Over eighteen-hundred letters came, in response to that follow-up article.

Some were from hurting moms and dads; some were from people who needed services for their handicapped child. Their letters were urgent and emotional and they all demanded answers.

We were incredibly busy—fulltime, nonstop!

# 8

It was well on toward ten o'clock one evening when I gingerly opened the door of Melissa's room. She sat huddled in the dark, head pressed against the crib slats, sucking her thumb and kicking her legs listlessly against the sides.

The moment she heard me, she uttered a delighted gasp and scrambled to her feet. I laughed and swooped her high in the air, kissing her again and again.

*I am so fiercely in love with this child of my heart, like none that went before. What savage passion reaches out to protect her, to shield her?*

Nothing would suffice but a rock together in the old maple rocker with Melissa cuddled in my arms. I sang, but there were no words, just a tune that roamed at will. Her monotone joined mine and together we hummed, off-key and sadly dissonant.

*The flesh of her arm is firm and hard. Is she indeed so far from normal? Is there really such a big difference, after all?*

A passing train whistled in the distance and the staccato of rain splattered noisily on the lawn umbrella on the patio underneath the window. I whispered funny noises in her ear to make the giggles come. And then, for no reason at all, a tear raced down my nose to drop on Melissa's upturned face. She stretched out a plump hand to touch the wetness.

*Oh, it's been so long since we've rocked like this, just slow and easy, as if we had all the time in the world. Mommy and Daddy are so busy. I'll bet you wonder where their strong arms are. But you listen, Melissa baby, you wait and see. We will show you something—something just for you!*

During this time of feeble beginnings, a most astounding thing happened. We had gone to pick up a chair that we had purchased from friends who were moving to Florida when, out of the blue, they announced that they would like to donate to Melmark the entire contents of their ten-room home: beds, chairs, mattresses, tables, draperies, TV sets, everything. We were overwhelmed!

And giving is contagious, for everyone likes to get in on the beginning of most anything. Starting something is exciting. So we had all the donations of material excesses that we could possibly handle. In fact, it began to be a problem to find room to store these things until such a time arrived that we could use them.

Our board of directors traipsed through "our" pink chateau the following week. They were unanimous in their approval. It would require a lot of tender loving care, but it was a good solid mansion built on seven inches of concrete under the first floor. The basement was a huge cavern with sturdy pillars of bricks and all kinds of mysterious wine cellars. We were thoroughly intrigued by all the possibilities.

Things began to happen fast. We were told that the owner of the pink chateau would accept an offer of $125,000 for the mansion and the surrounding twenty acres. She was willing to subdivide.

At our next board meeting, we signed an agreement to purchase the chateau in Newtown Square, Pennsylvania. Our realtor left for Philadelphia to procure the owner's signature on the dotted line. After everyone had left, Paul and I looked at each other.

"Tell me it's really happening," I begged Paul.

"It's true and it's happening."

"Don't tease me, Paul. It has been so long, I hardly have the faith left to think that we'll actually get any house, let alone this mansion that is so suited to our needs."

And just then, the phone rang. It was a lady from a local real estate office. She wondered if we were at all interested in selling our house, since about a year ago we had placed it on the market (that was back when we expected God to act fast and at our bidding).

"Yes, we certainly are interested. Just this moment we signed a purchase offer on a beautiful thirty-five-room home for Melmark in Newtown Square. Your timing is priceless!"

A family from Ohio was on the way over. We scurried through the house, setting things in order, telling each other that looking was one thing, buying was another, and not to get too excited. It probably wasn't going to happen this soon, anyway.

"Hey, kids, someone go answer the front door!"

About one hour after they had left, the realtor called with the breathless announcement that the family really wanted our home and they were willing to pay very near our asking price, but they wanted a ninety-day occupancy clause.

"No problem!" we laughed. But there was a problem, and a considerable one.

Andy, our realtor, came to the house that evening, and by the look on his face and the paper in his hand, we knew.

"Women!" And then he cast an apologetic look at me. "She wants $30,000 more or the whole deal is off."

"But, Andy, we just sold our house this afternoon. We have to move in ninety days."

"You aren't serious, are you?"

"We couldn't be more in earnest," Paul replied. "Right after you left, a realtor called to show a family from Cincinnati through our home. They liked it well enough to give us a down payment with a ninety-day occupancy clause in our agreement and that's about the size of it."

Andy just looked at us, somewhat stunned.

"But the other agreement was not signed by both parties yet." He was kind of softly sputtering.

"Andy, don't worry." Paul put his arm on his shoulder. "We are certain that this is the home that God has in mind for Melmark. And we are equally certain that he can provide another $30,000. That house is worth it. We'll poll the board and I'll let you know."

Paul was even then reaching for the phone. All the board members were in complete agreement. Just two short days later, we had the revised purchase offer signed by both parties with a ninety-day occupancy as well.

Now there were only two hurdles left. At least that was what our over-simplistic selves were reassuring us.

There was a zoning meeting that would decide whether the neighborhood would "tolerate" us, and then a mortgage commitment to be sought.

I had never been to a zoning meeting before. The long bare-walled room at the township building in Newtown Square was lined with folding chairs and rancid with the smell of stale cigars and cigarettes. It was already filling up with strange people, not one of whom I could recognize.

"What are they all here for?" I whispered to Paul.

"They are our neighbors." My blood turned to ice water. I fully expected them to take up placards and start marching around the room.

Near the front, we sat alongside our lawyer, By. Always, he was a quiet tower of strength and always, he was there when we needed him. He had his briefcase on the floor beside him and Paul had the rolled-up plans. I had nothing but pure panic.

I tried to size up the men who sat behind the wooden table stretched in front of us. They exchanged secret bits of intrigue, writing mysterious notes on papers on the desk. I wondered how we'd start this meeting. A hymn? Reading of the Bible? A salute to the flag?

The banging of the gavel seemed to be what they all were waiting for. Everyone stopped talking and I froze. I eased my tension by talking nonstop with God.

*Dear God, please stop to listen to me. These men have the fate of Melmark in their hands. They don't even know us. And our neighbors, all strangers, what are they going to say? Oh dear God, don't let them protest. Help them just to listen to what we are going to do. If they will only give us the chance. And God, stop my heart from pounding!*

Our lawyer talked about our plans and our motivation for establishing a home for the mentally handicapped. The supervisors asked many questions about the future. Then Paul was called up as president of the home. His drive and enthusiasm belied his forty-five years, in spite of the fact that his head was almost bald. And then, just like that, it was over. Paul sat down.

"Are there any questions from the floor?"

The male half of a charming young couple way in the back stood to his feet and said, "I am certain that most of our questions have been answered, Mr. Township Manager. We would just like to wish Mr. and Mrs. Krentel good success in their new venture."

I could have hugged him. And to this day, some twenty-one years later, he epitomizes the description of an ideal good neighbor. God bless the John Lyons of this world!

On May 27, 1966, my forty-fifth birthday, we moved into our pink chateau with volunteer help and a rented moving van, maneuvered inexpertly by our sons Bob and Steve. How they managed to get stuck under a railroad bridge on Swedesford Road, we did not discuss around the dinner table. At this point our family dinner table had expanded to include two Mennonite volunteer helpers, all of our own family (except Dave, who was married to dear Kathy and living in New York City) and our first three residents.

Moving day was a day to end all days. To be candid, my assignment in the center hall as director of traffic was the first big mistake.

"Take that to room No. 18. No, wait a minute, better move that to the third floor in No. 31. Oh dear, could you wait a second? I need to talk to Paul."

Just about collapsing time, women arrived from various churches looking like angels of mercy with hot coffee, sandwiches, and all kinds of calorie-laden cookies and cakes. That they did this every Saturday all through the summer will be forever to their credit.

Finally, the long hard day was over. Those who had the strength and good sense climbed the stairs and went to bed. Diane and Scubie slept on the second floor to watch over our three babies. Paul and I wandered aimlessly from room to room almost in a state of shock.

"We're here! We're really and truly here!"

"Well, it isn't what it's going to be some day, but it surely is a great start."

Up on the third floor, we surveyed the length of what someday would be our combination living-dining room and kitchen. It was almost forty-six feet long and boasted arched ceilings twelve feet high and dormer windows looking out on every side.

That night we simply dragged some pieces of furniture together, grouped them haphazardly around a portable TV, and that was "home" for the next six years.

When we finally slipped our weary bodies between the clean sheets, we sighed a huge inaudible prayer of thanksgiving. Long before the amen was reached, we had fallen off to a dreamless sleep.

Here we were, our own private worlds completely upended, blithely hanging the clammy reality of a $75,000 mortgage around our necks. Surely, I thought we must be mad!

And the publicity from my *Good Housekeeping* article gave us unprecedented exposure. Letters continued to flood in from parents seeking admission for their children—eighteen hundred letters in all!

One of our first admissions was Andy. When three-year-old Andy arrived, we learned what the true meaning of a "hyperactive stomach" was. It produced a condition called "rumination," a habit reminiscent of a contented cow. The one major difference was that the cow generally kept her mouth shut when partially-digested food rose from the stomach back to the mouth.

Andy was an exceptionally beautiful child, with curly blond hair and sable-brown eyes. But he was totally deaf and severely retarded, with hypertonic muscles and the distinct probability that he would never be able to walk.

It was well on toward midnight when his chic young mother had pulled up in a taxi in front of Melmark. She carried Andy, in his fashionable clothes, under one arm. After greetings were exchanged, she walked determinedly upstairs when I told her where Andy's crib was waiting.

"If you leave him alone, he'll go right off to sleep," she

assured us confidently as she departed in the taxi. "It's too late to go over all the details and I will see you first thing in the morning."

As I closed the big front door, Marilyn, one of our Mennonite service corps, was calling me over the bannister.

Two steps at a time, I made it breathlessly into his bedroom. Andy was nonchalantly standing on his head in the corner of his crib. Both feet were waving wildly in the air, and he was happily gurgling . . . or gargling.

"Hey Andy, what are you doing?" But he didn't even turn around. I had forgotten that he was deaf.

When eight-year-old Annie joined our Melmark family, her slim young father hefted her weight easily in his arms. But, when he sat down, Annie filled up his lap and spilled over the edges of the maroon lounge chair, her gaunt arms and spindly legs angling every which way awkwardly.

He sat there, wearily mopping his brow, and told me that he simply could not cope any longer. His wife had recently undergone heart surgery and Annie was becoming too heavy for her to lift or care for alone.

"We love her too much!" Large tears welled up in his brown eyes. And there it was, another heartache, packaged in slightly different wrappings. Color it tragic, all the same.

Annie arrived with three notebooks filled out by her mother with detailed instructions on "how to care for Annie." One concerned itself with "the only way to feed Annie." I could picture her mother-heart spilling out all her special little secrets to strangers who, she was no doubt convinced, would never care for Annie the way that she did. And I am sure we never did equal that life of devotion.

Now breakfast time became a distinct challenge. How fast could you get it into Andy before he started ruminating? How long would it take to feed Annie this time? And how much patience would be left for Terry, Todd, and Melissa, who by now were howling for more attention. It was a delicate balancing act, and usually the one who yowled the hardest got the most attention.

It also was a great aid to teaching self-help skills. The ones who could feed themselves were clearly better off. And it was amazing how quickly they imitated one another.

One thing that really bothered me in those early days was the unrealistic verbiage about retarded children. They were called God's special children, little angels who could do no wrong, each one exceptional and set apart. I often found myself wishing that whoever was circulating such high-sounding euphemisms would spend one day at Melmark.

Sure, the kids with Down syndrome were by and large easier to care for, but those boys and girls also had tempers, streaks of stubbornness, and unlovely qualities just like everyone else. And all of them, who fell in no one particular category, could make just the daily routines of life challenging. Sometimes we all got downright discouraged.

"It's Jo-jo again, Mrs. K. She's smeared her B.M. all over the bedroom wall." It was not pleasant scrubbing and scraping the wall for the umpteenth time that week.

And when big John came, we learned that perhaps the greatest humiliation can often occur while doing an act of kindness, like bending down to tie his shoes, only to receive a virtual shower of vomitus on your back.

It was no easy task, and sometimes childcare workers got discouraged and wanted to quit almost before they had started. It was one thing to change a baby's diapers, but quite another to deal with a twenty-two-year-old young man who had soiled himself.

Melmark was exacting its toll on our own Krentel family relationships as well. Too busy to write, too busy to phone, just plain too busy! We even forgot those special days . . . like birthdays.

# 9

On Diane's nineteenth birthday, she was away at Houghton College. Her boyfriend Ron took her out to dinner in a nearby restaurant. Much, much later she confided to me that she and Ron had had a serious talk that night.

"Did you hear from your folks?"

Diane shook her head.

"You mean they forgot your nineteenth birthday? I don't believe it, Dee. I'll bet there's a package or a card down at the post office."

But there was no mail and no telephone call later that evening. Diane, our incurable romantic, was hurting.

"They're so busy, they don't have time to think about birthdays. It's OK, Ron; I know they love me."

Ron kept silent.

"Besides, I can't wait until I see the completed renovations on that big mansion," Diane added. "I haven't even seen it. I can't wait! I hope they moved all my things in my bedroom. I wonder if I'll even have a bedroom of my own."

At the end of the month, when the time had come for Diane to come home for summer vacation, she was able to get a ride with a friend. When they pulled around the huge circle-eight driveway and stopped in front of the big mansion, Diane looked around for someone to greet her. But there was not a soul. The fellow who was driving unloaded her suitcases and left them at the front door.

Diane walked into the center hall. It was noisy and bustling with eager volunteers, not one of whom she knew. Standing on ladders and boards, paint brushes in hand, they were refurbishing the huge foyer.

"Does anyone here know where my mom is?" she asked of no one in particular.

Just then Bob came running down the front stairs and spotted her standing there. Leaving the suitcases, they both began to search me out. Upstairs, downstairs, asking everyone in sight, Diane almost despaired of any kind of a welcome home.

And then I spotted the two of them. The look on Diane's face was bewildered, like a little girl just waiting to be kissed and welcomed back to her family.

Tugging at the suitcases, we helped her up to our third floor apartment. As yet, we had no door to our apartment that would shut out the busy world and allow us to gather together as a family. This was a hidden cost that we hadn't considered when starting up something as time-consuming and demanding as Melmark.

The next evening, when I was almost too weary to hear what she was saying, she chattered on and on about her new love, Ron. Then she commented that she noticed that many of the staff at Melmark were calling me "Mom." I hadn't thought about it; it just seemed to be sort of natural.

"Do you mind, Dee?"

"Sometimes," she admitted. "You're not their mother—you're mine!"

I understood her fierce protectiveness. There was simply no private Krentel world anymore. The walls had all come tumbling down and we shared our meals, our laughter, and our special family times with our childcare staff and volunteers.

I must admit there was no hiding place. And now even Diane was trying to guard the last crumbling bulwarks of our family life. It must have seemed like an impossible task.

All that summer, Diane and Scubie performed their childcare duties with all their young vigor. This even included working the dreaded night shift, when the huge mansion just sat there in the foreboding darkness, hugging its history close and daring the most recent occupants to make new memories.

It was scary making those rounds when everyone else was sleeping. The steps creaked and the walls groaned and even crackled in seeming protest at our presence. Two bedrooms on the east side of the second floor now sported new colors of orange and green painted on huge polka dots which Paul pasted up on the ceiling. The bathrooms gurgled at all the water rushing down its pipes and protested the frequency with which it was called to tolerate this humiliation.

Ladybird, our family collie, was enlisted to escort the night duty staff on their evening bed checks, but after a few good-natured steps, she lay down and adamantly refused to move, despite all of Diane's coaxings.

A fire check had to be made throughout the cellar which, at that time, was an endless series of concrete caves. A huge hissing steam boiler supplied all our heat and hot water, much too willingly.

That first summer of beginnings was long and hot.

Our new daughter-in-law Kathy, with B.S. and R.N. degrees from Columbia, served as our first head nurse while David, our firstborn, commuted to his job in Philadelphia.

We all cooked, ate, and worked together as family—staff and babies and Krentels—all summer long. It was small wonder that our own family relationships were a bit strained.

David and Kathy had not as yet celebrated their first year of marriage. And Kathy, looking like a shiny version of Florence Nightingale with her long dark hair, sky-blue eyes, and freshly starched uniform, was all we could ever want or need for our head nurse.

Kathy's head was simply spinning with creative ideas just waiting to be tried out. And Melmark was ready to try them all, for this was a family project. There was no red tape to be cut before a decision could be reached.

Melmark received the full impact of her post-grad fervor. It went far beyond her nursing duties, varying in scope from staff scheduling, menu-making, and medications to ordering of new cribs and picking out new uniforms for our childcare workers.

Before long, David, her new husband and our eldest son, began to feel that perhaps he was taking second place.

One hot midnight, Paul and I quietly left the big house to take a dip in the swimming pool by ourselves. The air was almost too oppressive and stifling to breathe. We walked

64

through the remains of the formal gardens, swung back the iron gate, and went down another set of granite steps leading to the pool.

In the dim light, at the deep end of the pool, we saw a lone figure sitting on a green wooden bench.

"Well, Dave! Great! Are you going in swimming?" Paul called. "Where's our Kath?"

"No, I'm not going in now. And Kathy is doing tonight what she does almost every other night: either making out schedules or planning new menus."

"Hey, I'm sorry, Dave, I didn't know. Is there anything we can do to help?"

"No, it's not Kathy that needs the help—it's me. She loves it and I guess I'll recover."

We were growing so fast. We had really not anticipated that God would bless our efforts so promptly. What had innocently started out as strictly a family affair, now grew unpredictably and in all directions. And each one of the family pitched in wherever the need was the most pressing.

In those early days, I was the chief cook and bottle washer in addition to interviewing new applicants and parents of children who needed a home like Melmark. Often I looked into the eyes of parents so weary and worn from day-in-day-out care of severely involved children, that my heart would almost break.

I will not soon forget one battle-scarred father who came to Melmark to find a place for his son. I can almost see his face as he talked to me. His manner was aggressive, and it was clear that he had hurt for a long while over his son. Suddenly he got up from his chair and said,

"Do you want to see my son? He's out in the station wagon. Or do you only care for the cute little ones with Down syndrome?"

We walked together out to his car. Throwing open the back door of the station wagon, he defiantly watched my face as I looked at his son lying on the back seat of the car on a blanket. He was an older boy with rough stubble on his face, his body covered with open sores and red pimples. Curled into a tight fetal position, he did not even open up his eyes. Inwardly, I recoiled; outwardly, I tried to control my facial expression as I reached out to stroke his head. It was difficult to find a place that was free from open ulcers. But I knew I must touch him.

"We have a very young staff," I offered, as an opener.

"And you don't think they could tolerate the looks of my son. That's it, isn't it?"

I swallowed hard and tried to speak.

"That's OK," he said. "I don't know why I expected this home to be any different. I'll throw him away in some garbage can somewhere; then nobody will have to look at him."

He got in his car, slammed the door, and drove away. It took quite a few minutes to regain enough composure to get back in the house. Today, I am still haunted by the tragic defeat of that meeting and my inability to reach out to share this poor man's burden. It is a haunting memory, some twenty years later, and I often wonder what happened to that helpless boy.

Almost before we knew it, the summer was over, Diane returned to Houghton, and soon it would be time for David and Kathy to leave for Texas. David planned to study for the ministry at Dallas Theological Seminary. Our farewells were teary, for we had grown so interdependent. We simply did not feel quite able to swim without their encouragement. And we worried about what we would ever do for a head nurse!

But God was always one step ahead of us.

Fran, a young registered nurse, with experience in the field, applied for the opening. Later, she laughingly confided that God did not lead her to Melmark—he pushed her!

"When three people hand you an article saying, 'You must read this,' and, 'perhaps here is a place that needs someone like you,' what are you going to do?"

And for the next five years, until she left for Zambia as a missionary, she served the children of Melmark loyally and capably.

Bob attended Eastern College while working parttime in physical education in one of Pennsylvania's largest (and most prestigious) private schools for the emotionally disturbed and mentally retarded.

Melissa had opened up his eyes to the world of the handicapped, and he grasped every opportunity to learn more about their special needs. But more importantly, he was getting priceless experience working with the handicapped, experience which we would later use at Melmark.

In those first few months, Bob was certainly used of God to bolster up our woeful lack of exposure to this needy group.

# 10

I don't think I will ever forget the day we accepted Mary Lynn from Massachusetts. Drawn to us through the *Good Housekeeping* article, Mary Lynn's mother had written a letter which was a masterpiece of sorrow interwoven with personal victory. Both parents were tired out and battle weary; they had sacrificed much in the way of a normal family life over the years.

When Mary Lynn arrived at Melmark, our first brief conversation took place in the driveway. Her parents mumbled their friendly greetings hurriedly, as they tried to coax Mary Lynn from the car. It was clear that they wanted to present themselves as a family. I looked the other way and waited.

Hearing the sound of metal chains rattling, the very wildest of thoughts careened through my mind. When I permitted myself to look again, my eyes widened at the size and the sight of Mary Lynn—a tall big-boned girl with fear-struck eyes, shaking a length of metal chain in both hands, and jerking her head back and forth. Close-cropped auburn hair whipped against her face as she soundlessly communicated a message to her parents. She was clearly not going to get out of the car!

"Sometimes things that are metallic make the best toys," her mother explained cheerfully. "I found this little chain on a discarded purse of mine, and Mary Lynn loves it." We both laughed nervously.

At long last, they convinced her, by a combination of yanking and pushing, to step out of the car. In the center hallway Mary Lynn squatted down on the floor and refused to budge, uttering sounds that were a cross between a horse's whinny and a run-down siren. I was petrified and trying very hard not to show it. A Down syndrome baby was one thing, but this was clearly out of my sphere. Whatever dedication or altruistic motives I thought I possessed were quickly getting smothered.

Around the dinner table, I confided my fears.

"I can't tell what she's thinking or what she's going to do next. I don't know how to handle her, or, frankly, even if I want to learn how."

Bob spoke up quickly. "Listen, Mom, she's like a lot of the kids where I work. You have to get to know her; then you will like her. You'll begin to discover what all her little noises mean. Remember, she's trying to communicate with you."

I was only slightly comforted. The next day was Sunday, and I was determined to go it on my own. I had prayed about my attitude and decided that God certainly could not accomplish one single thing through me until I became personally involved with her. So I volunteered to take care of her.

I fed lunch and dinner that day to Mary Lynn. Each time I swooped the spoon toward her mouth, she deliberately looked away.

"Now, see here Mary Lynn, we can't throw away all this nice dinner. And I'm only trying to help you, OK? But you must look at me. I can't find your mouth, so you will have to help me."

We got through dinner, somehow, with her genteel parents discreetly waiting in the center hall. Then we went for a walk outside. That, her parents had told me, was one of her favorite activities. But if what I had in mind was a brisk, arm-swinging walk around the driveway, that was clearly not what Mary Lynn had in mind. So I matched her footsteps. First, we shuffled a few steps, then hesitated, then took a few mincing steps, and, once in a great while, a few normal strides.

Most of this time she looked steadfastly away from me. It was clear she was sizing me up. I don't know what gave me the courage, but the second time around, I grabbed Mary Lynn by the waist, and we hopped and skipped to my boisterous singing: "Here we go loop-de-la, here we go loop-de-lay." Suddenly she stopped, grabbed me around the neck in the crook of her left arm, and whinnied loud and long into my left ear. I stared at her, almost mesmerized by her face right next to mine. Then

I reached over and quietly kissed her on her smooth cheek. I could hardly wait until Bob got home from work that night.

"You wouldn't believe it, Bob. She, well, she is different and she has very interesting little ways of trying to communicate. But you know something? I think I like her!"

Monday mornings were always the hardest, when Paul drove off to work in Philadelphia, leaving me in charge.

This was the first real business experience I had ever had. I loved it, but I was completely unorthodox and a bit casual in my business proceedings.

Paul, coming home at night, weary from his Philadelphia commute, was forced to hear my endless accounts of everything that had occurred that day at Melmark.

I wondered how long he would be able to stand the stress of working two jobs, for that was exactly what he was doing. All of the unfinished business that so badly needed his administrative capabilities was there waiting for him at Melmark after he had already put in a full day's work at his job in Philadelphia.

We talked long and often about the possibility of making it without his pay check. By the first of October, we could stand it no longer, and Paul resigned. Now there were no more commuter trains to catch, no briefcases to pack—just work, work, work, sixteen hours a day, then drop off to sleep, painfully aware of the challenges and the burden right underneath our third-floor bedroom.

Wake up the next morning, roll out of bed, and head downstairs to the office. And there it was, waiting for us, all over again.

There were adjustments. Some were Paul's: when the telephone rang and people asked for Mrs. Krentel; some were mine: I had to relinquish some authority as he began to take over the reins. It took me a while to find my true niche. But oh, Melmark was so much better off!

One morning I heard Melissa cry. Her bedroom was right under our kitchen. She cried for the longest time, and it was all I could do not to run down to comfort her. I listened for some signs of lessening grief, but she continued to sob, a despairing wail. Finally I could stand it no longer. Reaching for the intercom, I called the nurses' station.

"Did Melissa fall and hurt herself?"

Head nurse Fran knew what I was asking. So often there was no need for words between us.

"I'll go check, Mrs. K. Call you right back!"

I waited, straining every fiber of discipline within me. I had battled this one before, and the victory seemed to come and go. It was not always easy to be right there and watch someone else doing all the things that I, as a mother, wanted to be doing for my own child. And I recognized that many times it must not have been easy for those who were caring for Melissa, with her mom and dad somewhere nearby.

Fran didn't call back. Instead she popped in at our apartment.

"Just thought you might have a second cup of coffee for me," she smiled. "Melissa pushed Debbie, and Debbie cut her lip, so Melissa was put back in her crib, away from the other children."

"Thanks, Fran." I poured out two cups, hot and steaming, the aroma satisfying.

In my comings and goings at Melmark, I frequently saw Melissa with five or six other toddlers. I always stopped to hug or kiss my small daughter, but lately I had noticed that an imperceptible change was taking place, a small but hurtful change. I no longer was the "king pin" in Melissa's life. Her meals and baths and fun times all were taking place and I wasn't even on the scene.

So it seemed that gradually I was relegated to the role of an "extra." Melissa now greets me with the enthusiasm and charm that she accords any casual passerby. And, although it might seem odd, I cannot bring myself to single out Melissa from the rest of the group and grant her all of the special favors that my mother-heart cries out to give to her.

Besides, even if I wanted to, it isn't physically possible, for whenever I walk into the Orange Room I am immediately swarmed by Melissa's roommates. Everyone talks at once, clamoring for attention, sitting on my lap, and asking to go "Up, up, Mommy Krentel?"

They have figured out exactly where I live: the third floor of Melmark. So, most of the time, when Melissa climbs up the stairs to our apartment, she has Amy, Charlie, Terry, Billy, or Debbie in tow.

What can I say about that day when our hearts were stolen by a five-year-old? When Rodney first visited Melmark, he was accompanied by a county social worker. Earlier that week, Paul had received a phone call from Bill, in charge of placements for Montgomery County. Bill challenged Paul with a "highly unusual case" which needed a residential setting such as Melmark. This would be not only a "highly appropriate placement" but one which would, in his opinion, greatly benefit his client.

Two days later, a sturdy boy not quite five years old arrived at Melmark with a somewhat hesitant social worker in tow. Paul and I met them in the center hall. We walked outside together to the front driveway.

Rodney did not say one word, nor was it necessary. One look from his bewildered brown eyes and I would gladly have bartered my inheritance to win his affection.

The weather was beautiful, the kind of a day that every May day should aspire to be. I laid my hand lightly on Rodney's shoulder and asked his caseworker what kind of timing they had in mind for the boy's admission to Melmark.

"Today." The word hung there, hopefully. "He's staying in a hospital bed," she explained, "and there is no medical reason to support that kind of placement. Three foster homes have not been able to manage him, you know." She added: "Belligerent attitude, destructive behavior."

I looked down at Rodney.

"Why don't you go and take a look at our play yard," Paul suggested, guiding him gently toward the swings.

It took her a moment before she resumed her mechanical recitation. Rodney was happily swinging, out of earshot. "This whole case is pretty dismal. We do not seem able to find a foster home that is able to meet the needs of this child. His parents are separated and the mother does not want to take care of her children. He is almost five and is unable to say

72

many words. He has a language age of eighteen to twenty-four months and relies on grunts and gestures for the most part in communicating his needs. He has an IQ of sixty-seven and is hyperactive and aggressive toward other children."

She paused for a moment as Rodney had tired of swinging and had returned to join us. He looked up at me with a most lopsided disarming smile.

Paul reached over and grabbed my hand. I squeezed his fingers. It was as though we held a quick meeting of the Admissions Committee right there in the circular drive.

"Well," he smiled, "I think we may be able to find room for this fine boy. Yes, we'd love to have him come to Melmark."

The case worker lit a cigarette.

"I trust it will work out for you and that he won't cause you any trouble."

In addition to all the challenges and problems that marked the beginnings of Melmark, love and romance were blossoming all around us. Ron was wooing our Diane, Bob was courting Ruth, and Roger and Scubie were an "awesome twosome."

It was difficult, at best, to hold those special little family gatherings and keep them private. Everything seemed to be public knowledge often before we were even informed. Good humor seemed to be the most essential ingredient in keeping peace.

Whenever flowers arrived at the front door at Melmark, the news traveled swiftly. Everybody seemed to know about it long before Diane did. And when her fiance Ron arrived from Syracuse to visit her, the event was heralded by phone and intercom and young staff running up to the third floor.

Bob moved up his wedding date, from June to March. The entire family was pleased, for we all were in love with his Ruthie. It was good to get our minds off of Melmark. We preened like peacocks in our wedding finery as we left for church from the center hall.

But there was no personal privacy. Everything we did attracted intense scrutiny from the Melmark residents. The only way into or out of our apartment was through the girls' hall. And sometimes it seemed that they just were waiting for us to pass through so that they could find out where we were going and how long we would be out.

"Going for a walk" could be construed as going to Florida for a vacation. Coming back upstairs to a chorus of "Did you have a good time, Mommy Krentel?" often served as a harsh irritant. Sometimes we wished we could be invisible, simply to reach our third-floor apartment without comment.

And then it was time for another wedding; this time it was our daughter Diane. And she was most anxious that we do it right, but she loved every detail of the pre-wedding planning.

The day of the wedding dawned hot and humid. It was right in the middle of an August heat wave. The photographer took many wedding pictures in the center hall in front of the big mirror and down the lovely winding staircase. Staff and students alike enjoyed the colorful spectacle. Melissa said over and over, "Dee-dee, pret-tee!" It turned out to be a storybook wedding.

Then, quite without warning, we entered another season of our lives, one in which our parents suddenly expressed needs which often accompany "growing older," needs which they thought we could meet. So just when we thought our nest would soon be empty, it started to fill up again.

Steve was living at home while attending Brandywine College and our family expanded to once again include him. My parents, Grandma and Grandpa White, came to live with us at Melmark and again our family circle grew.

Since we lived on one end of the third floor, we put a door at the other end of the hall and made another apartment for my parents: a little kitchen, a bathroom, and a small living room.

It seemed ideal . . . or so we thought.

# 11

Bright and early one Saturday morning, Paul and I drove down to Lankenau Hospital for X rays to be taken of Paul's gallbladder. I think the unknown troubled us more than we cared to admit. I was certain it was ulcers and, in the back of my mind, I was worrying about cancer. Paul's father had died at fifty-two from stomach cancer.

We sat there in the hospital hallway. Somber faceless people garbed in the anonymity of pale green hospital gowns were vacantly staring at nothing. It was a cheerless sight. There was little chitchat.

After the X rays, one of the nurses came over to us. Paul stood to his feet.

"Go home and get a little breakfast, Mr. Krentel. The doctor will call you with the results."

The phone rang about two hours later. It was the doctor.

"Your gallbladder, Mr. Krentel, is one solid stone. I think we need to talk about an operation."

Paul's face sagged as he relayed the news to me.

The phone rang again, even as we sat there discussing this new problem. This time, however, it was our son-in-law Ron. I don't think I will ever forget what he told us. His voice was guardedly jubilant. They had been waiting for what had seemed a lifetime to Diane—three-and-one-half years—to finally begin their family.

"Mom, we have a beautiful little baby boy, named Matthew Ronald, and he weighed in at seven pounds and six ounces. . . ."

I let out a very unladylike war whoop.

"Only one small problem . . ." his voice trailed off, and I did not believe I was hearing correctly. The words were very matter-of-fact. "He has a small opening at the base of his spine, but nothing to worry about, Mom. They are going to operate on him over at Memorial Hospital. So we think that everything should be just fine."

I did not ask any questions, for suddenly it dawned on me that the condition he was describing was spina bifida.

"We'll be there as soon as we can catch a plane, Ron."

Hastily, we threw some clothes in a suitcase and raced for the airport.

It was a one-hour flight. We arrived in Syracuse just as they were getting ready to wheel Diane out of the delivery room. We threw our arms around each other and wept. I was not completely sure why Diane was crying, but I wept with pure, unadulterated grief.

"I'm a mother, Mom! I'm finally a mother! Can you believe it? Matthew will be just fine!"

We walked back to the small private room where Diane proceeded to give us all a detailed account of the birth of Matthew. She babbled on and on happily. It seemed to Paul and me as we stood there listening that she either did not know, or was not facing up to, the full implications of this "little hole at the base of his spine."

*Where is her doctor?*

Neither one of us could find the proper words. Finally, the pediatrician came in. He was amazingly detached as he explained what this birth defect was all about. And I could see Diane's eyes widen in alarm. He mentioned the fact that attempts at repairing the hole would involve more than one operation. One would involve a shunt to drain fluid from Matthew's head to his stomach.

It suddenly hit Diane. She knew from her Melmark experience what a shunt was.

"You mean my baby's going to be . . . retarded?" Her voice was shrill and hysterical and my heart bled for her. Paul stood there obviously distraught. This was his oldest daughter, his Dee-dee. Ron stood helplessly by her side holding her hand. There was nothing any of us could do but stand there. The full impact of the doctor's pronouncement hit us all full force.

When the doctor left, we tried to console her. But all she

could think of was this nightmare end to her beautiful dream.

"Mother," Diane sobbed, "why would God do this? Why, oh why, would he ask us to go through a Martha, a Melissa, *and* a Mattie? How could he do such a thing?"

I did not know, nor would I even pretend to fathom what God was doing with the Krentel family. I knew one thing, though: my mother's heart was shattered with grief for my own daughter. I was discovering that standing on the sidelines and watching your loved one suffer was far more difficult than going through it firsthand.

Later that evening when visiting hours were over, Paul and Ron left. Diane begged me not to go home: "Mom, I don't want to be alone. Will you stay all night with me?"

We shoved two green arm chairs together, face to face, and it looked like a good enough bed for a very short person. We laughed about it briefly and the nurses obliged by giving me a pillow and light hospital blanket.

Then that long night began. Diane was in high gear and needed to talk. And I needed to listen, to understand the scope and depth of her pain.

"Mom, I noticed right away, right after I had given birth, that my baby's cry was not real strong. The doctor said that I had given birth to a baby boy. But the most awful thing, Mom: they whisked him right away. And I just lay there on the table. Oh Mom, I just had this awful feeling that Mattie was dead; I couldn't hear him," she cried.

I did not say anything, for I knew it all would have to come out. My own eyes were brimming.

"And Mom . . . nobody talked to me. I kept asking, 'What's wrong? Why isn't my baby crying?' And finally one of the nurses came over to me and just grabbed my hand and squeezed it real hard. I'll never forget the way she said it. Oh Mom, it tore me up. She said it so quietly: 'Diane, your baby has a birth defect; he has spina bifida.' I remember saying something dumb like, 'Spina difida? What is that?' She explained that it meant a divided spine, which sometimes leaves an opening on the base of his spine. Mom, I had the impression by what they said that he would be OK from the waist up but his legs might be paralyzed. And I know that sometimes paralysis and mental retardation go hand in hand."

I was listening hard and praying even harder.

"Can you believe it? I've given birth to a baby and they wouldn't even let me hold him in my arms. Mom, you know what? I think he's dead and they won't tell me. Mom, did you see him? Has he gone already over to Memorial?"

Diane closed her eyes. And we both were very quiet. Minutes later, she reached over and grabbed my hand.

"Mom, you'll never believe what's happening to me. Each time I close my eyes, all I can hear are the words to 'The Lord Is My Light.' Do you remember that song? We used to sing it in glee club. It's Psalm 27."

Taking out my small pocket Bible, I began to read it and Diane and I both found comfort and inner peace in those promises.

Five days later, Diane came home with empty arms. Ron did what he could to comfort her, but all the new furniture in the nursery reminded her afresh of her little one left behind in the hospital.

Operation followed operation during the next several weeks. "How long are they going to experiment on my baby? Is anything really going to change his condition?"

Matthew also had the Arnold Chiarri syndrome. Our precious little grandson kept forgetting to breathe and had to be placed in a special incubator which buzzed an alarm to remind him to inhale.

Seven weeks of the most exquisite torture followed. The nurses were kind. Some would encourage Diane by phoning her to say that he seemed better on that morning, or the doctor would inform them of some new test that might prove to be the breakthrough.

They visited him every day, yet the only way that they could hold him in their arms was when they were garbed in sterilized green gowns and white masks. And even in their arms, he was connected by wires to some machine. Once in a great while they were allowed to feed him his bottle. Diane had always planned to breastfeed, so this was added trauma.

Then, just when they felt as if they could no longer endure

their seesaw emotions, little seven-week-old Mattie died. He weighed three pounds and four ounces.

There was a private burial service in the rural cemetery for baby Matthew two days later. The morning of the graveside service, all of the family were together again in Ron and Diane's small cottage by the side of Lake Oneida. The skies were leaden.

Diane's eyes were red and puffy. She sat close to her Ronnie in a big lounge chair in the living room. Abruptly, Diane stood up and went over to the stereo, put a tape on, and turned up the volume. The Wheaton College Men's Glee Club was singing, and we all interrupted our sorrow to listen to the words.

> We praise Thee now, O God
> With hearts and songs and voices!

We bowed our heads. I think it must have gladdened the heart of God to see his children still praising him with bursting hearts in the midst of their trauma. His ways are past our finding out.

*Tragedy is so swift, so unannounced. It catches me off guard, defenses down, helpless as a newborn, open to each onslaught, until at last I cry out: "You win. The battle is over. Pick up the remnants of my life and leave. I give up!"*

*And, precisely at that moment of my surrender, the soothing balm of Christ within begins the healing process: calming the turbulent waters, mending the heart strings, fixing my open sores, my empty heart, the torment of my mind, until at last I can feel the faint stirrings of hope working again the miracle of peace and joy in the midst of all the havoc that tragedy wreaks.*

Interwoven with these distressing family circumstances were the problems of our growing family of handicapped at Melmark. I kept a personal diary of some of these early heartaches. One of the editors at *Good Housekeeping* encouraged me to keep on with my writing. I was challenged to do so, admittedly, but there seemed to be precious little time for the writing about the growing pains of our home that love built.

But in spite of time limitations I managed to write the first five chapters of a book about Melmark. Finally, one day, I read in one of my writer's magazines that there was a contest for "a nonfiction book that demonstrates the strength of Christian faith in a contemporary world."

Fantastic, I thought! God placed me in the middle of a book; all I needed was discipline—a simple enough request.

It took four weeks to complete the next fifteen chapters. I scribbled on a yellow legal pad and Mary, who had come to Melmark as a result of my magazine articles, typed it over at night. Finally we managed to get it all together. I sent it out to the publishing house, not daring to hope too hard.

Back it came, three months later, rejected despite making it through the first cut. Having invested my heart and soul in the writing of it, I did not feel like doing much more with it. So I sent it off in the mail, unrevised, to Moody Press in Chicago.

The good news of their acceptance was reward enough for some of those grueling nights. Finally we had a written history of the birthing of Melmark: *Melissa Comes Home.* I was thrilled that God was using whatever talent he had given me to communicate to others who were hurting.

When at long last the published book arrived, I caressed the shiny cover, turning it over and over in my excited hands. It was the most beautiful book in the world to me! And it seemed to open new doors of ministry for me. I began to receive invitations to share the story of Martha, Melissa, and Melmark.

I will not soon forget one such speaking tour. I was heady with excitement as I packed my suitcase and piled four cartons of my new book in the back of the station wagon.

This would be a great opportunity to speak for Christ, and a wonderful way to publicize Melmark. The entire four-day route was arranged so that the meetings were well within easy traveling range.

I was scheduled to speak at eight women's luncheons and dinners. The noonday occasions were for the mothers, and the evening for career and professional women. Sponsored by a nationally known women's group in California, the meetings were to be held mostly in the state of New York. Overnight accommodations were arranged in various sponsors' homes.

80

I planned to sell copies of the book after speaking, using their book tables. These groups were quite accustomed to such a practice, exhibiting many religious books, paperbacks, and other items that might interest women.

It was different traveling alone. I had never been away without Paul or the kids. Arriving in Binghamton for my first speaking assignment just fifteen minutes before they were ready to sit down, I was greeted by a friendly hostess who escorted me to the head table.

Wending our way through the ladies, buzzing with happy conversation, the president of the club spotted my tote bag filled with *Melissa Comes Home*. She murmured something indistinctly.

"Oh yes," I hazarded a guess, "just where do you want me to put these?"

She was visibly flustered as a faint pink crept to her cheeks. I hadn't the foggiest notion what was bothering her.

"I really don't know exactly how to say this, Mildred. But I received a call from headquarters just this morning telling me that our club would not be allowed to sell *Melissa Comes Home* on our book tables."

"Why not?" I was dumbfounded.

"Oh, I know it's just a beautiful story. I cried all the way through. But we have an editorial committee who must approve any written material that we sell. And your book . . . your book does not have the plan of salvation in it." She stopped, too embarrassed to go on.

"Well," I explained, "it really wasn't written as anything but a chronicle of a Christian pilgrim going through some of the darker valleys of life. It was simply intended to be a witness of God's faithfulness to his children."

"I know, I know! But we do have to abide by the rules from headquarters." She was talking a bit louder now.

My head was swimming. They could trust me enough to speak before all these women without the faintest clue of what I was going to say or how I was going to say it. And yet they refused to allow my book to be sold.

My mouth felt like cotton, though I spoke firmly, "I understand that you always have a backup speaker ready in case your speaker does not show. Isn't that true?"

"Why yes, but . . . but, what are you saying?"

"Simply this: since what I am verbally sharing with your group this noon is all written right here in my book, then I am afraid I will have to say that my book and I go together. Both of us . . . or none!"

She was visibly flustered. We stood there looking at one another. The room was a beehive of finely-dressed women completely unaware of the little drama being enacted in front of them. She looked up at me and smiled tentatively.

"Well, we want you to speak; that's why so many of these women came. We have over three hundred reservations today."

"Look," she hesitated a little moment, "I'll take the responsibility; let's do it. It doesn't make a terrific lot of sense to me either."

BOOK BANNED IN BINGHAMTON! I could almost see the headlines screaming. I was crushed. I felt like starting for home right after this luncheon and let their headquarters cancel the rest of my speaking schedule. I don't know how I managed to speak, because my heart was beating double time. After I spoke, the books sold like hotcakes. Some of the women even came out to the station wagon to get more.

*Have I not measured up to someone's understanding of what a Christian should be? What exactly constitutes a Christian book?*

I called Paul from the home of my hostess, as soon as I placed my suitcase in my room. He was as unhappy about my predicament as I was.

"I'm going to turn around and come home, Paul. Maybe I shouldn't have come on this silly trip."

"It is not a silly trip. You went to share your Christian faith, and now the devil is doing whatever he can to keep you from doing just that. Don't get discouraged. I can get in touch with their headquarters. You just wait there and I will see if I can find someone to clear up this mess."

I went upstairs to lie down on the bed. Taking off my high heels, I waited for about an hour. Then, at long last, the phone rang. It was the founder of this national group of clubs. He spoke lovingly and sweetly, but his honeyed tones only served to irritate me more. His tone was precise and his reasoning inflexible. He was quietly adamant about the decision.

"Next time you write a book, you should include the ABC's of the plan of salvation."

I stood there, hanging on to the receiver, feeling like a fool, blowing my nose and weeping.

"Let's pray together, dear, shall we?"

"No, thanks," I managed to squeeze out, "I'd rather pray by myself."

When I hung up, I literally ran back upstairs into my quiet little room. There was no sound from below and I really did not know exactly what to do. I was scheduled to speak that evening at a dinner for business and professional women.

Feeling that it was not a good testimony to walk away from the whole situation, I decided to meet my commitments. I would simply tuck one or two books in my brief case, just in case someone from the audience wished to purchase a copy.

That evening, with the air of an undercover agent, I mentioned offhandedly the publishing of my new book. I sold both books and took orders for ten more.

The remaining engagements for the week were well attended. God blessed in spite of me and my horrendous attitude. By midweek, I carried my tote bag full of books again.

Nobody said a word. Whether or not the judgment from California had reached the ears of the chairwomen up and down New York State, I do not know to this day.

I was beyond caring.

# 12

One early morning as I lay in bed, I heard a most persistent noise. Could it possibly be someone knocking at the door of our third-floor apartment?

"I'm coming!" I yelled none-too-gently. I pushed away the warm blankets and grabbed my husband's slippers and robe as I opened the door to our haven of rest. A nineteen-year-old childcare worker named Debbie stood in the long hall, looking as if she would burst into tears at any moment. Her pinstriped uniform and starched cap seemed inappropriate backdrops for her panic-stricken eyes.

"It's Marylou again!" she blurted out.

"Where now?"

"Under her bed. I can't get her to budge. All the other girls are downstairs eating breakfast."

"I'll handle it." The words came out with reassuring calm. In no way did they indicate my inner state of being. I belted up my husband's extra-large bathrobe and shuffled down the hall in his size-twelve slippers. Debbie was bouncing along the hall with a vigor fairly nauseating at that hour of the morning. I peered at my wrist. Without my glasses, I could barely see the watch, let alone the numbers.

"6:45, Mrs. K.," Debbie volunteered.

I groaned.

Marylou was flat on her belly under her bed. The pink flowered bedspread was a gypsy tent. As soon as she spotted my feet, she turned her myopic blue eyes toward the wall.

I squatted down on the floor and threw back a corner of the bedspread. Marylou did not move. Her strawberry-colored hair floated around her milky-white face, thick-lensed glasses hesitated halfway down her nose, and her spindly arms and legs bore little resemblance to her chunky body.

She lay there, thumb in her mouth and fingers stroking her nose. It was difficult to remember that she was sixteen years old. Yet her application had stated it bluntly, adding rather succinctly, "This child is subnormal in intelligence."

"Good morning, Marylou."

She eyed me suspiciously.

"Hey, move over a bit." I nudged her playfully.

She managed to squeeze out an inch or so of space for me. I maneuvered alongside her awkwardly.

"This is a great hiding place! Didn't mind my coming in, did you?"

"Nope!"

"What happened to upset you, Marylou?"

"I'm mad!"

I asked the question she was obviously waiting to hear next: "What made you so mad?"

"My honey-bunny—she went away."

"Well, nobody told me. She's the best helper we have around here—just about," I amended, lest she quote me later on.

"Her didn't even say goodbye!"

"You must be teasing me."

"Nope!" As soon as the words were out of her mouth, her thumb was back in.

"Well, I don't exactly blame you for getting all upset. Hey, let's get out of here. It's getting hot. Let's talk about it!" In the confusion of squirming out from under the bed, I managed to lose one size-twelve slipper, but, since forward progress was being made, I decided this was not the time to retrieve slippers.

Five minutes later, Marylou had clarified the reason for her discontent. Her very favorite childcare worker, Mary, had not been on duty in the girls' wing for the past four days. I deduced that Mary must have been assigned to the night shift and was probably fast asleep by now. But Marylou was not prepared to accept what she clearly regarded as a lame excuse. Suddenly I jumped to my feet, grabbed both her hands, and dragged her upstairs to the third-floor staff area outside our apartment.

"Wait and see; I'll show you something," I whispered, with the air of a conspirator. I softly turned the doorknob to Mary's bedroom, letting Marylou peek through the crack. The moment she spotted that familiar dark head wedged into the hump of her pillow, a foolish grin crept over Marylou's face.

I pulled the door shut quietly, and together, hand in hand, we walked down the stairs to breakfast. At the door of the dining room, she left me happily and took her place around one of the small formica-topped tables.

There were about twenty boys and girls seated around five tables. You might have thought you had stumbled into a high-school cafeteria. But, if you lingered a moment, you would have heard the babble of half-finished sentences, the unexplained laughter, the siren of an ascending scream; you might have seen the unblinking stares, the greedy attention paid anything edible, the unabashed thievery of loose morsels of food.

Debbie looked up briefly, spotted Marylou seated complacently in her chair, and gave me a big wink. She continued to place heaping spoonfuls of scrambled eggs alongside buttered slices of toast. One of our Mennonite workers deftly served it with one hand while whisking over-sized terrycloth bibs from the fireplace mantle with the other. She tapped my shoulder and pointed wordlessly to a football helmet resting on the floor by the chair of a thin-faced boy of ten. His protruding cheekbones were covered with self-inflicted purplish welts and bruises. I nodded and walked over to pat Bobby on the shoulder.

"Good boy, Bobby. You don't need your helmet, after all, do you?"

He threw me a penetrating look.

"Daddy . . . will . . . come . . . in . . . the . . . morning."

"Well," I hedged, "probably not until the weekend, Bob, but it won't be long."

"Morning . . . bells . . . are . . . ringing," he chanted, his voice an insistent singsong.

A few of the older girls had noticed me and started to giggle behind their hands as they observed my unusual attire. I acknowledged them with a sweeping bow, holding my red plaid robe regally around me, as I flounced out of sight with a hasty goodbye. My precipitous exit only brought me headlong into the path of an advancing battalion of eight toddlers on the front stairs heading for their own special mess hall. Shepherded by a diminutive Miss Lottie, they step-by-stepped down the winding carpeted stairway, hands clinging to the leather-wrapped balustrade.

And then I spotted Melissa. She had planted herself dead center on the stairs a good five steps higher than where I was and had prepared to fling herself in my general direction. I had no sooner braced myself than my arms were full of my five-year-old mischievous little Down Syndrome daughter.

I wiped her nose on a big white hankie I found stuffed in my husband's pocket. While I smothered her with kisses, she patted me on the shoulder somewhat condescendingly. And then, just as quickly, she was off, blowing me kisses and heading for her first love—oatmeal!

I pulled out the hankie again.

Life seemed to continue in a vicious cycle. We no sooner lost a member of the family, than we would birth another one. Rodney, from the outset, seemed destined to be a true member of the Krentel family. Steve commuted to nearby Brandywine College and also worked at Melmark. It was not long before he too had fallen victim to Rodney's charms, and his innocent query, "Up, up?"

Big Steve would scoop up Rodney and arrive upstairs with the little guy clasped in his arms. As we delighted in the progress in Rodney's speech, Steve asked if we would mind if Rodney moved in with him and shared his bedroom.

"You know, Mom, he really needs the extra challenge we could offer him."

So the following memo was sent to all staff: "Rodney Horner has transferred his sleeping quarters to the third-floor Krentel apartment. This move has been made with specific parental approval in an effort to increase his verbalization to the point where he can successfully communicate in any environment."

Rodney loved being special and he grew by leaps and bounds. Soon he was learning to substitute "I" for the "me" that had started out each and every sentence. He would say, "Me no like it, Mommie," while the cooked vegetables grew cold and pasty on his plate.

Around the dinner table, we devised a "penny" game. For every time that Rodney said "I" instead of "me" we would give him a penny. But if he made a mistake, he would forfeit one of his pennies. He loved the game and we finally succeeded in eliminating the incorrect use of the personal pronoun. (Highly unorthodox means to an end!)

We were in the midst of a blinding snowstorm. Driven by a steady northeast wind, the snow was powdery and fine—a magnificent display of God's artistry, yet somewhat frightening to Paul and me. We worried whether or not our live-in staff could continue their childcare duties until our commuting relief staff could make it in.

Melmark's plow made little impression on our roads and driveways. The snow blanketed the cars parked in front of the Main House and rested heavily on the branches of some of our loveliest firs. Many trees surrendered without a protest. Limbs crashed to the whitened ground with muffled sighs.

We fretted about milk deliveries and did-we-have-enough-oil, for we were isolated at the end of a deadend street. And the roads had not yet been opened. Everybody was trapped in a white, white world where the weather clearly had the upper hand. Those who sought to fight the elements lost the battle—some sooner, some later.

Early on the third morning, we were still snowbound. We had not run out of supplies, but everyone was dead-tired from working almost all shifts. Bob was working the plow, trying to clear the side road so that we could reach Route 252 and pick up some relief staff. Many could not even make it out of their own driveways.

That was the morning that Paul decided to get outside and help Bob with the plowing. The weather was brutally cold. I couldn't even read the thermometer; it was all iced over.

Paul bundled up, downed a steaming cup of coffee, and, with muffler over his mouth, left our apartment to brave the elements. Walking out the front door, he noted that it was not

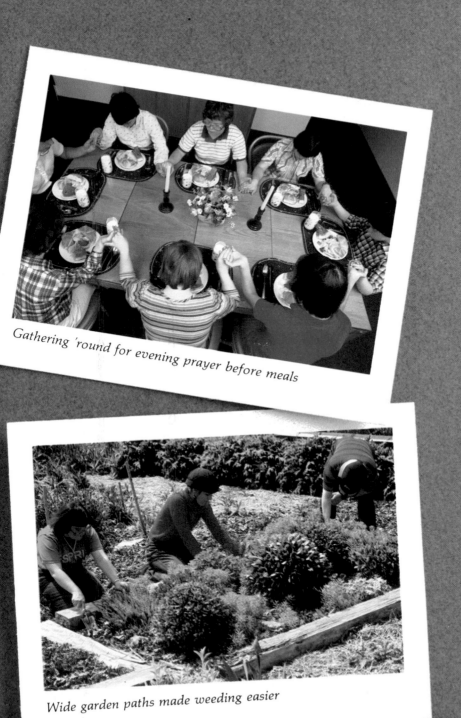

Gathering 'round for evening prayer before meals

Wide garden paths made weeding easier

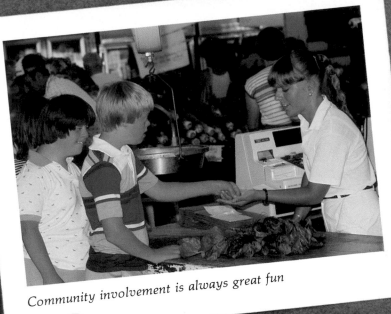

Community involvement is always great fun

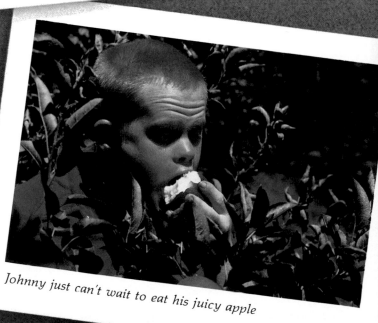

Johnny just can't wait to eat his juicy apple

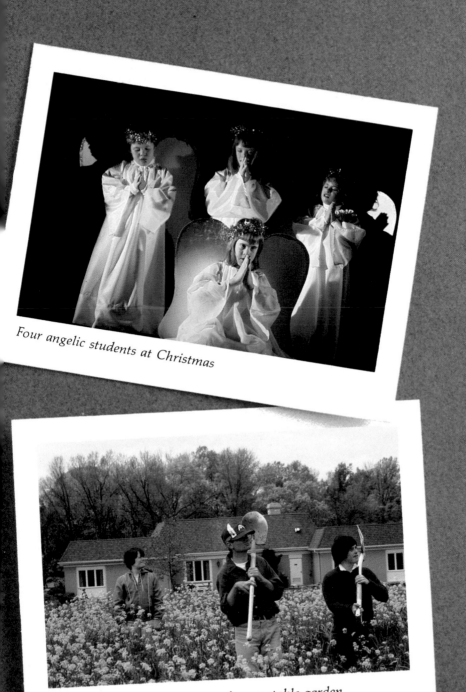

Four angelic students at Christmas

Melmark students enroute to the vegetable garden

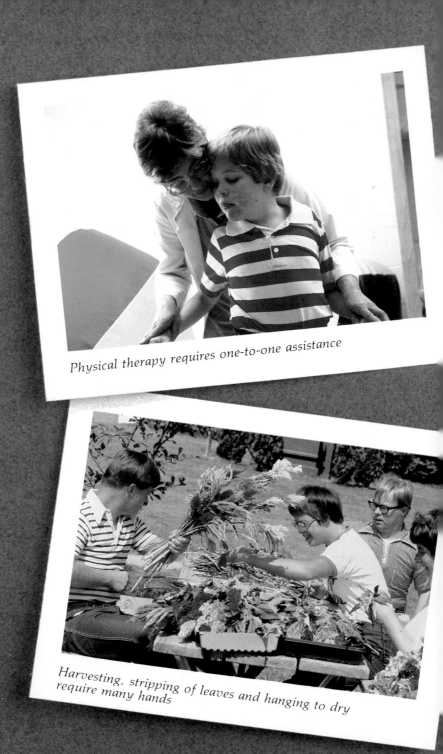

Physical therapy requires one-to-one assistance

Harvesting, stripping of leaves and hanging to dry require many hands

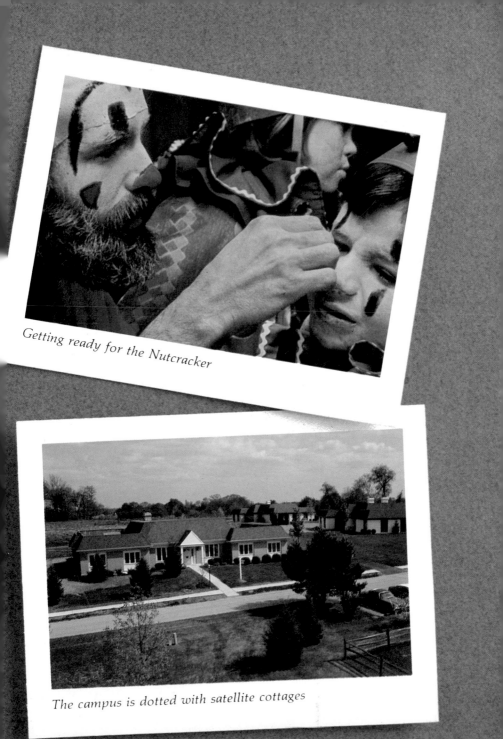

Getting ready for the Nutcracker

The campus is dotted with satellite cottages

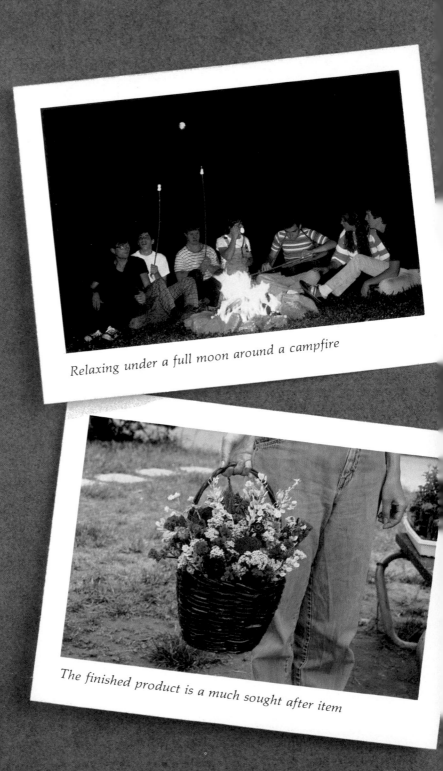

Relaxing under a full moon around a campfire

The finished product is a much sought after item

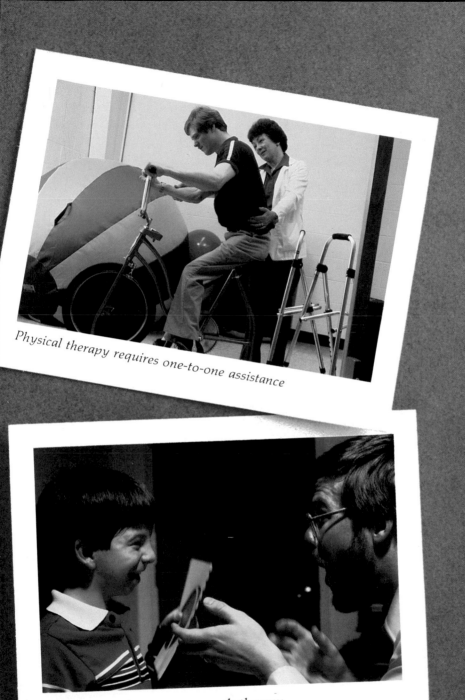

Physical therapy requires one-to-one assistance

Language development or speech therapy
need enthusiasm

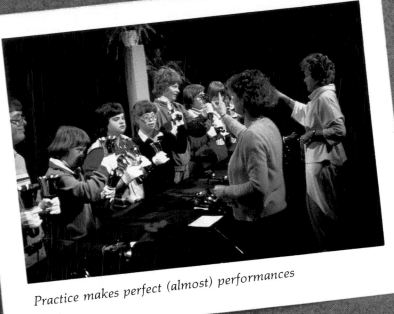

Practice makes perfect (almost) performances

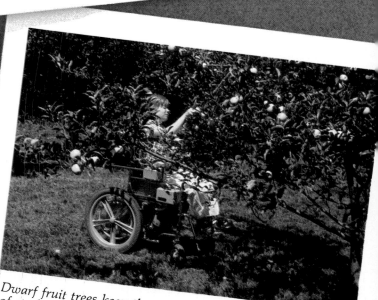

Dwarf fruit trees keep the apples within easy reach of students in wheelchairs quite seven o'clock. Many of our residents were still sleeping soundly. Carefully he picked his way over to the side stairs leading to the lower level parking lot. He held on to the banister and made it gingerly all the way down safely.

Then, as he walked over toward the jeep, his foot slipped on an icy foot print in the snow. Down he went, a tremendous pain shooting through his body.

Paul couldn't move. He bellowed and roared like a bull, but nobody was out or about to hear him. I was upstairs, blissfully drinking that second cup of coffee.

Twenty minutes passed and no one heard his calling. The white quiet was almost mesmerizing.

Suddenly Paul heard the sound of the side door being pushed open with a shove. Again he yelled as loud as he could, and heard the answering voice of Ginny, one of our nurses. Paul kept on yelling so she could find him.

"I think I broke my hip," he grimaced with pain.

"Oh, I'm so sorry. Don't move, Mr. K. We'll get you warmed up until an ambulance can take you to the hospital," Ginny said soothingly.

Blankets and newspapers were brought to keep him warm, and the ambulance was called. Paul's teeth were chattering and I was afraid that he was going to go into shock. But he kept talking and remained conscious for the agonizing two hours that it took for the ambulance to get to Melmark.

Then, when we arrived at the hospital, we discovered that his doctor was also snowbound. The X rays confirmed a broken right hip; his two frost-bitten buttocks confirmed the fact that he had lain in a snow-filled driveway for over two hours.

Two weeks in the hospital and a slow recovery time were sufficient reminders of the blizzard of '72!

# 13

Ⅰt was a giant step of faith and we did not take it lightly. Our growth pattern developed from a base of need. We simply could not stand still.

For over five years, we tried to keep pace with our population explosion. During the first year of operation, we enclosed two porches and remodeled five small rooms in which we had been housing resident staff. That gave us room for fifteen more residents. In the second year, we added a nursery and a sunshine room for multiply-handicapped persons.

Our Melmark family grew to ninety-one, all residing in one thirty-five-room French chateau built in 1914. We ate in shifts; we took turns in the big playroom. We improvised at making classrooms where there were none and transforming unused space into needed bathrooms. It was mind boggling but challenging.

We had discovered that our Melmark family responded to a varied program of stimulating physical and educational activities. Water therapy had proved to be of great benefit to our physically-handicapped boys and girls.

During the summer months, it was easy. We conducted swimming classes in our two outdoor pools and used our playground and tennis courts to their fullest. But summer is short and there were nine long months when the swimming pool was all covered up and the weather was cold and uninviting. We realized that we would have to expand again in order to stretch the horizons of the physical, mental, and spiritual worlds of our limited children.

One Saturday in February proved to be a red-letter day in Melmark's history. After an all-day meeting with our board of directors, it was voted unanimously to approve a $1.13 million building project. Plans were made to proceed full speed ahead with a gymnasium, swimming pool, three cottage-type units to house forty-five more children, and two new staff residences.

On a sunny May afternoon, a year later, Melissa, Todd, and Terry, the first three residents of Melmark, grabbed the big handles of the gold-painted shovels and did their best to dig in the rocky earth. It seemed fitting that these little ones who had tangled themselves up so completely in our hearts and lives should be the first ones to break ground for the new construction.

It was a simple ceremony. The trees stood tall and proud where the new cottages would nestle, the sun shone brightly, and the wind blew in playful little gusts. We prayed, and even Melissa bowed her head. We sang, and the people that had gathered there for this momentous occasion joined with us.

Praise him, praise him,
All ye little children,
God is love, God is love!

Soon the bulldozers arrived, and in the sloping hillside a nesting place was hollowed out for another outreach, another arm of the home that love built.

After eleven months of building activity, our Dedication Day was upon us. The weather was delightful, an unseasonably balmy April Sunday afternoon.

"Come and share in our happiness," the invitations read. And come they did! Nearly one thousand people crowded into the new gymnasium-auditorium. We were humbly awestruck, as they packed the aisles and crowded the doorways, straining their ears to catch every word. Many stood outside the doors, unable to find standing room inside.

It was a heartwarming dedicatory address delivered by Dr. James Boice, pastor of Philadelphia's Tenth Presbyterian Church. He used the text from Exodus 4:11: "Who maketh the deaf, the dumb, the seeing or the blind. Have not I, the Lord?"

A simple program was presented by Melmark's own children. There were rhythmic interpretations by the kindergartners, the first public performance of the Melmark handbell ringers, and two vocal solos. The audience lent enthusiastic applause, punctuated with occasional indulgent laughter at the inevitable mix-ups of any children's program.

Four-year-old Debbie, a Down syndrome little girl, struck a responsive chord when she sang, "There were six little ducks sitting in the water," with appropriate impish actions.

Twelve-year-old Gary, a microcephalic boy, limped haltingly to the front holding his one twisted hand awkwardly with the other, his brown eyes serious and unblinking behind his tortoise-rimmed glasses. He quietly stood, looking over the crowd, waiting for the simple piano introduction. Right on pitch, he sang in a clear boy-soprano voice.

Only believe, only believe,
All things are possible, only believe.

Each word came out distinctly enunciated, a credit to Melmark's speech therapist. There was not a dry eye left in the audience.

Then, Allen, our resident "pastor-painter-houseparent," came forward and offered a heartfelt prayer of dedication, after which Dottie, his wife, sang, "Bless this house, O Lord, we pray."

And suddenly it was all over. The overflow crowd stood to its feet to tour the new facilities and partake of the refreshments served by the gracious Melmark Service League. Paul and I stood up at the front of the gym in the doorway, and shook hands . . . for two hours!

I couldn't believe this miracle was happening. Our visitors "ooh-ed" and "ah-ed" over the ramped indoor swimming pool, the physical therapy room, the showers and lockers. They marveled at the cottage wing which included three separate living units embodying the then-popular "family-living" concept. This wing provided room for forty-five more children.

It was a day never to be forgotten, for it marked the beginning of a new life for our children.

*It is too much, God; we are breathless! But that's kind of the way you do things. You are an over-and-abundant God, never stopping halfway, never thinking that things need not be so special for the "least of these." Our hearts are full to brimming with great thanksgiving. Thank you, dear God, thank you!*

About this time in Melmark happenings, our youngest son, Steve, had fallen head-over-heels in love with his college sweetheart, Trish. Soon another storybook wedding took place.

Sometimes events seemed to play tag with one another in their eagerness to find a place in our lives. Summer and winter seemed to follow right after one another on our busy calendars.

Somehow Christmas mornings were the best. Since our family had always opened gifts on Christmas Eve, it was easy for us to adjust to spending Christmas morning with those boys and girls at Melmark who did not go home. The tree was laden and the presents spread over the floor in the center hall at Melmark.

It was festive and fun to share in their happiness. At mid-morning, the boys and girls gathered—some creeping on the floor, some running down the long hall to the Main House, some drag racing in wheelchairs, childcare workers with their arms full of those who couldn't make it on their own. Many of the staff, not even supposed to be working on Christmas, were there helping everyone get dressed and fed.

While we waited for the slower ones to arrive, Pop-pop led the singing of "Jingle Bells" and then "Joy to the World." (Everyone, from the youngest to the oldest, called Paul "Pop-pop." It was a comfortable and appropriate name that somehow fit his role in their lives.) Each Christmas, he would look around at the diversified group, many of whom could not talk or walk, and he would ask the same question that he asked every Christmas: "And whose birthday is it today?"

The responses were loud and barely recognizable. But it made no difference; Pop-pop knew the answer too.

"Jesus!"

Then we prayed, thanking God for all of our blessings, and sang, "Happy Birthday, dear Jesus." Many Christmas mornings it took almost two hours to open all the presents.

Once again our home was enlarged with "growing older" parents. Now we had to consider their problems, facing their future as well as ours. This time it was Paul's mother. After

Paul's stepfather died, his mother declared that she could not keep up a home so far away from her family. So Mom Rix sold everything and moved back east to live with her daughter in New York.

Then, the grass always being greener somewhere else, she decided to come to share an apartment with my mother. Since Father White had died, it looked like an ideal arrangement for both of them.

By this time, Paul and I had moved from our third-floor apartment into a separate staff residence on the Melmark campus. So, Mother White and Mom Rix took their places in our spacious former apartment in the Main House.

They seemed happy as two bugs in a rug, entertaining the Monday morning group of volunteers and baking molasses cookies and Swedish coffeecake. We thought all our problems were solved. But whoever said life would be simple?

Troubles broke out on our home front; this time it was Rodney, who had inched his way into the heart of our family. He had been living with us for almost five years and was making excellent progress. He accompanied us on vacations, enjoying holidays and fun times.

Rodney was now attending public school. He was in a special education class and rode the school bus. One day he arrived home from school, visibly upset.

"Kids on the bus . . . they call me . . . retard!"

Hot, angry tears accompanied this accusation. My heart went out to him. What could I say to assuage his shame?

"Rodney, I'm sorry. I really am!"

It was not a situation that we could control. I tried out the old adage about "sticks and stones" to give him psychological insulation from his peers, but it was a long, hard struggle.

Academically he was making fairly good strides. But his inability to read fluently hindered his forward movement. He handled mathematics but any material that had to be read and comprehended slowed him to a grinding halt. In addition to lacking reading skills, Rodney wasn't getting along in school. He was fighting on the playground and was unruly in class, especially when lessons beyond his grasp were given.

I thought perhaps a status report on his behavior at the end of each day would keep some of these problems from becoming overwhelming. At least we would be able to reinforce at home the teacher's efforts at school.

I could always tell when Rodney had not fared well. His round cheeks became a deep red. His brown eyes nearly popped with brightness as he tried to make me understand what he was going through. My heart cried out for him, but I could not help him.

One day, a particularly distressing event occurred. Rodney had run out the side door of the classroom and dashed clear around the school building. By the time the teacher caught him, he was hot and flushed. He squirmed out of her grasp and ran to hide in the boys' washroom. The teacher was not to be denied and ran after him. Standing in the doorway, she spotted Rodney sitting on the tile floor in the far corner. He was sputtering and spewing out some choice four-letter words and included her in some obscene accusations.

When he finally stopped, she told him to go to the principal's office—whereupon, I was called to pick him up. Rodney had been suspended from school for three days.

We were saddened at this turn in his behavior. He was reverting to the behavior that had expelled him from three foster homes prior to his arrival at Melmark when he was only five years old. We did not know which way to turn. Clearly something drastic had to be done before it was everlastingly too late.

We thought about alternative schooling arrangements. We knew he needed the special education that would enable him to function in society. So we talked with one of our board members who was Director of Education of a very fine educational institution, where we were finally able to make suitable arrangements for Rodney. We planned to enroll him as a day student in a school which specialized in his kind of problem.

That weekend, I drove him to his home to visit his mother and siblings. We had stopped to buy a dozen doughnuts for his small brothers and sister. Standing there at the front door of a row house, we waited to be let in. The sound of running steps and the barking of a puppy indicated someone had heard. The door was flung open with a bang.

I stood in the living room and watched Rodney's brothers and sister descend on the doughnuts with abandon. Rodney's mother came down and we stood and talked in the living room while the children spread white sugar and doughnut crumbs all over the floor. Rodney tried to get them to take the box of doughnuts to the kitchen, but nobody was listening. He looked at me and shrugged his shoulders.

I told Rodney's mother what Paul and I had in mind for Rodney's schooling, to see if she were willing to go along with this new plan. Without warning she began to cry, her voice picking up speed, volume, and pitch as the discussion progressed.

"You can't have my son. He's mine. You have no right!"

"Listen, please," I said softly. "I don't need another son; I have three of my own. I'm only trying to help Rodney."

"I want him home with me; I don't want him to stay with you." She wouldn't look at me.

"I didn't bring his clothes," I offered hesitantly.

"You can bring them another day."

She was adamant. It was all over. I knew the final curtain was crashing down. I walked over to Rodney, who gazed at me with a helpless look of love. I threw my arms around him and he put his head down on my shoulder. He never said one word. And I walked out alone to the car.

I never again heard from Rodney or his mother. When enough time had passed for healing to have taken place, I tried to locate him. But the row houses had been torn down and I discovered from a neighbor that his family had moved to Reading.

*I wonder what Rodney looks like now. How is he faring? Does he still remember us?*

It certainly was one of the more painful experiences in our life at Melmark.

# 14

Contrary to our expectations, and for no apparent reason, Paul's mother and mine began to argue over the most inconsequential things. Tears and angry accusations flew back and forth.

Both were such refined ladies that we found this new development difficult to deal with. Maybe it was a sign of approaching senility. Whatever the cause, we had to confront the problem and make some drastic changes in their living arrangements.

One fog-filled day, I put the question to Mom Rix: "Would you like to move in with us? Would it be any easier for you?" My own mother was much too independent even to think of that alternative, so it had to be Paul's mother who would move.

I dreaded her answer, because I almost knew what it was going to be. It came, a quiet, defeated, guiltridden, "Why that might be nice, dear—if you really want me. I wouldn't make any trouble for you or get in your way."

So Mom Rix moved in with us. We thought this change of environment would surely help. And Mom Rix was ever so careful not to disagree or argue, because we might ask her to leave and live elsewhere. Then, where would she go? Whatever would she do?

Since I worked every day at Melmark in the Main House, I carefully provided lunch for her in my absence. Mom insisted that I must not worry. But the more she insisted, the more I worried.

Soon, I discovered that the soup I had left for lunch was scorched on the bottom of my heaviest pan. The tea kettle had burned dry, the bottom melting on the burner.

97

Mom Rix, always my tower of strength in the past, was crumbling to a pillar of salt before my eyes. I vacillated between resentment and guilt. I resented the intrusion that caring for her made on my own life, and I resented the time it took away from my husband. I felt guilt about these resentments and at the stark realization that I was certainly not the loving daughter-in-law that I once thought I was.

Mom frequently cried at all the trouble that she felt she was causing. She hated being alone all day, but she hated our big Great Pyrenees dog even more. She would not let the dog stay in the house, but pushed him firmly down the cellar stairs the minute I left home, whereupon he rewarded her by incessant barking and scratching at the cellar door.

Table talk ceased to have any relevance. Mom got the past all tangled up with the present. Unrelated verbal minutiae became almost intolerable to hear much less to make any sense of.

It was then that television news and game shows took the place of dinner conversations. Talking was only resumed during the commercials. Then Mom would look up at us brightly, like some expectant bird, and offer inappropriate comments after our telegraphic attempts at communication.

The situation worsened. Telephone messages were garbled or undelivered. One day, I came home a bit later than usual. It was pitch black as I fumbled for my keys, silently begging the dog to stop yelping, please. And there lay Mom Rix, on the floor. She had fallen and could not get up. She could give no coherent explanation as to how long she had been there. There were no bruises, no bones broken, just bruised pride and broken spirits.

The conversations about what to do about Mom Rix ran long and hard in the refuge of our bedroom. We had to find a proper nursing home to take over where we were failing.

We finally located one place that could offer Mom a reasonable facsimile of her present lifestyle. Looking it over carefully, we found a corner room that we could furnish to her taste. She would be able to walk down the hall to the dining room, where all the ladies partook of their meals together.

Next came the biggest question of all: Would Mom accept this as a viable alternative? We skirted the issue carefully, gingerly touching the subject now and again and just as quickly changing the subject before she could comment negatively. When we finally popped the question, Mom, surprisingly enough, agreed to at least look at the home.

It was a big afternoon. We arrived, with Mom looking her happiest. She greeted everyone she saw, waving cheerily. We sat down and talked to the executive director of the home and Mom promptly launched her campaign by coyly suggesting that maybe they would not admit her.

The director then suggested that maybe as long as she was there would she like to go down and meet their medical director. The director was enchanted with our charming octogenarian and had concluded that she would make a delightful addition to their home.

So we went down to the medical director's office. He was very young, making a studied attempt to be casually aloof and professional. After listening to her heart, he posed a few questions.

"Well, hello there, and how do you feel?"

"With my fingers!" Mom answered pertly.

He looked at her rather blankly.

"And how old are you?"

"Old enough to know better," came the quick reply. He gave her a wan smile, and I laughed awkwardly, trying to make him see the humor in the situation.

"Can you tell me what date it is today?"

"My goodness, I never can keep track of the days, they come and go so quickly."

"What is your husband's name?"

"Which one?" He looked bewildered and disgruntled.

"Mom's first husband died." I offered quietly, certain that she would never pass muster.

"Where do you live?"

"With Mildred and Paul." This she was sure of.

"And where is that?" he continued, doggedly.

"Oh, wherever they go, I just go right along."

"What is our President's name?"

Mom looked at me, puzzled, and waited for me to answer. I did not dare. Finally after a hard silence, I broke into a cheerless laugh.

"You know, Mother: Jimmy. . . Jimmy. . ."

"Jimmy whooo?" she asked good-naturedly. It was of no use.

He gave up all attempts at conversation and took her blood pressure. After thumping her dispiritedly on her back once or twice he said, "You can take her back upstairs now."

I knew she had flunked. There was no way that they would accept her as an alert, contributing member of their home's population. We walked back upstairs quietly, my heart heavy.

Driving home, Mom chatted incessantly about all the friends that she could have at the home. It was a real turnabout, since we had assumed that she had had no intention of moving.

In a few days, the director called back with the news that she had "passed" her physical and that the doctor had noted "senility and a mild forgetfulness" on her chart.

When we told Mom, she was elated. And we were overcome with guilt. Was this the happy solution that it seemed to be?

*This must be what the parents of Melmark's residents feel when they leave their loved ones in our care. It certainly isn't easy. I really have the best of both worlds. Although Melissa is at Melmark, Melissa is also at home with Paul and me.*

The day finally came when she was to be admitted. It was the third of July. We had feverishly shopped for her room, purchasing a special rocking chair, matching bedspread and curtains, teacups and new plants. Her room looked charming and, when we left her that evening, Mom patted us on the shoulder and said, "Well, I'll see you tomorrow at the Fourth of July picnic."

We came the next day and she shone! The morning star now had no competition. We visited Mom faithfully every Sunday, rarely finding her in her room when we arrived. She was off playing the piano in one of the many small living rooms. Visits were pleasant. She never asked to come home or questioned us as to how long would she be staying there. She just seemed to accept the home as a new part of her life.

But nothing lasts forever or stays the same for long. Mom fell in the hallway one night at the home and fractured her pelvis. From that point on, she was confined to her bed. Her descent was rapid.

One Sunday, when we arrived at the nursing home, the director met us. "Your mother just passed away some thirty minutes ago. We tried to call you but you were on your way here."

The funeral was simple, with two of our sons taking part. The grandchildren sang, "Jesus loves me," and Melissa joined in with her off-key enthusiasm.

Melissa looked at Mom Rix lying there so peacefully in her casket and shook her head sadly back and forth. We have tried not to shield Melissa from the various ingredients that make up life: the sorrows, the joys, the arguing that sometimes disrupts a family, the disappointments, the delays, and even the deaths.

Melissa knew where Grand-mom Rix was: "Up in heaven," she would point confidently.

From a "mustard seed" beginning, our Melmark family had grown to include 143 boys and girls. And we stood once again on the threshold of another building program. This time we planned for three satellite cottages to accommodate students in a "least restrictive environment" and another cottage that we called The Pines, to house some multiply-involved boys and girls.

It was a giant step of faith which would cost well over $1,000,000. But it was another step of faith that the needs of our growing-older family dictated that we make. Our educational programs needed to change to keep pace with their diverse needs.

We had left behind our babies somewhere during this incredible growth process, for they had grown up into mischievous, noisy youngsters of ten, eleven, and twelve, climbing, running, learning, and making each day a bit more challenging—and frustrating!

During this time of Melmark's growth, the Krentel family underwent what could have permanently fractured our circle of family love.

Family-run businesses are not all chocolate layer cakes. Relationships can often be confusing. And role-swapping—from boss to father to husband—is not all that easy. When does the business day end? Why is it that business discussions go on from sunup to sundown, around the dinner table, to steal away the fun and fellowship we all so badly needed as a family? Talk of Melmark even invaded the magic of pillow talk.

We resented it, but we seemed powerless to escape its grip over us. Melmark captivated our every move, smothering our outside activities and friendships until everything and everybody seemed to revolve around Melmark.

Bob, our second eldest son, worked side by side with us, sharing the weals and woes of our extended family life. We had weathered many an emotional storm in our first ten years. Problems were anticipated, if not always welcomed.

But, clearly, we did not expect them to linger in our own family. We had always prided ourselves on keeping short accounts, which meant simply that if either of us said or did something that caused hurt, we would be just as quick to ask forgiveness.

But then one day I felt as though our world had stopped. Bob walked into Paul's office and nervously, but emphatically, stated that he was going to have to leave Melmark. Nothing could have prepared us for that moment.

Quietly he explained that he had to leave to prove to himself that he could make it on his own in the world without riding on his father's coattails. Paul depended on Bob greatly. His work was beyond reproach and he had grown to shoulder more and more of the burdensome tasks that accompanied Melmark.

Bob stood there, his face grim and ashen. His blue eyes were troubled and he found it difficult to get out the words. But his message was all too clear. Paul with blanched face, tried to dissuade him.

Three weeks later, we watched their family pack up and go: Bob and his precious Ruth, and the children, Scott and Julie. A cloud of desolation swept over us. That night, the moon was full and shone in our living room, where two rocking chairs faced the window. We sat in the dark and turned on the stereo to play a Gaither recording. The words ministered to our broken hearts.

> Hold on, my child,
> Joy comes in the morning,
> The darkest hour
> Is just before the dawn.

As we rocked, we wept as though our hearts would break. It was not a decision that we could understand. We felt as though a divorce had taken place in our family. Why would God let this awful thing happen?

We discovered that healing takes place over a passing of time. This is most necessary. The hours, days, and months need to flow beneath the bridge and we must hang on, until the murky waters begin to clear and peace comes.

In the meantime, the Krentel family was still intact. Ruth and Bob never compromised their expressions of love toward us. For that we were most grateful. But, I must admit, there was still that stone of hurt on the bottom of my heart. I did not bid it welcome, but it insisted on taking up residence.

*Where can I go to heal a broken heart?*

# 15

Standing in the wings offstage, I could scarcely believe the thunderous ovation our Melmark Joybells were receiving. They were grinning from ear to ear, the girls curtsying and the young men bowing. All the pride of accomplishment was theirs and they felt ten feet tall!

I leaned against the pile of tables at the back of the stage and remembered the genesis of Melmark's bell choir. That beginning was so long ago. It started out simply.

Christmas was coming! Along with Christmas, came the need for a Christmas program presented by students for their parents. But what could our Melmark residents do that would be worthy to be called a program?

A play was out of the question; a singing choir would be disastrous. There seemed to be but one avenue open, or so it seemed to me that very first Christmas: a bell choir.

I purchased a small set of resonator bells for the sum of $7.98. Carefully covering each bell with different colored foil, I directed "Joy to the World" by pointing to a colored chart with a pencil. Even the audience recognized the tune.

It was a beginning, but clearly not a satisfying one. The bells simply were not of good quality. In our next *Melmark Messenger* I included the following ad:

SO THE BELLS MAY CHIME

We are seeking one set of eighteen chromatic hand-tuned Swiss bells. When this equipment is finally located, Melmark will be able to include a Swiss Bell Choir as part of its child development program.

Somebody out there was listening. A business executive in New York City sent a check for $500. And we discovered that some of the most beautiful handbells in the world were made in Sellersville, Pennsylvania. We visited the Schulmerich facility and soon we were the proud owners of a two-octave set of bronze handbells. Very carefully, I picked out fourteen boys and girls to try out for our first bell choir.

They did not have to be able to read music in order to make this musical contribution—most of the original fourteen could not even read. There was no musical talent involved other than rhythm, and no more important requirement than immediate obedience to a given command.

And from that simplest of all beginnings has developed a touring choir of twelve boys and girls who call themselves the Joybells. They have played on television, at the White House, twice for Governor Thornburg's inauguration, and have been invited to Jerusalem to play at the International Assembly of Choirs.

It never ceases to amaze me that this group of twelve handicapped young people have enormous appeal to audiences of all ages. Perhaps it is their disarming guilelessness and rapt attention that catch audiences off guard.

Clearly, it is a two-way blessing! Wherever they go, they make an undeniable statement that their lives, no matter how limited, have a right to be lived to the fullest.

Our invitation to play at the White House came about as a result of an unsolicited letter, written to the wife of the President of the United States.

> Dear Mrs. Reagan,
>
> I would like to take this opportunity to say thank you for your public stand against abortion. It takes great courage to openly and freely state one's beliefs, especially when one is in, or associated with, public office and your belief is in opposition to many of the vocal public. I salute your courage.
>
> There are many ways that courage is expressed. The one that stands out most in my mind at this time is the courage it takes to live with the results of standing by one's principles.
>
> This holds true especially when those principles involve the very essence of life and death. And death

is what the proponents of abortion on demand would have for any child that might possibly be born with a physical or mental handicap.

I have recently come in contact with a group of retarded young people who have been spared the executioner's medical procedures. These boys and girls are residents of the Melmark Home for the mentally handicapped in Berwyn, Pennsylvania. I met them in the course of their tour of churches across this great country of ours.

These children have Down syndrome, yet their birth defect has not prevented them from being accomplished handbell musicians. Their music is inspiring and audiences are filled with admiration for them.

In their eyes, the height of accomplishment would be to perform at the White House, if a performance could be possible. I respectfully request that an invitation be extended to them. Perhaps this could give hope to many people with handicapped children and stem the tide on the abortion issue.

Sincerely,
Paul Samuels

Yes, we did play for the Christmas party of the executive staff and their families. Watching our President and his wife walking down the stairs to greet the people gathered there on that festive occasion was so exciting; it was a topic of conversation for weeks afterward.

The Joybells now have four octaves and a three-octave set of hand chimes. They are able to play handbell music very much as it is written. Two directors lead the choir—one each for bass and treble. Use of sign language will eventually allow us to use only one director.

Celia Downie, Melmark's music therapist, explains how sign language is used to direct the choir.

Playing in a handbell choir is an ideal way for handicapped individuals to express themselves musically. Bells are simple to play and provide a great way to learn through group participation. The Joybells are such a group, playing together for the Lord.

A person first seeing the Joybells perform may wonder how it is done. At first glance, it seems complicated. The ringers stand behind the bell tables with four (sometimes five) bells assigned to each person. Their attention is intense as they watch the two directors wave their arms, sometimes pointing, sometimes making funny little fists, in front of the long bell tables where the bells rest when not in use.

Actually, the whole process is quite simple. The bells are set up like a piano keyboard. The two directors stand in front of the table and point or signal the individual bells as if they were the keys of the piano. When more than one bell has to be played (that is, a chord), the director must rely on the visual cue, perhaps one finger, or two, three, or four, held up to designate a particular chord.

These particular cues trigger the ringer's memory as to which bell to play. When more difficult passages of music containing many chords in a sequence occur, a technique, in which we utilize sign language, is used. The method is unique, and, as far as we know, originated with the Melmark Joybells.

Sign language simplifies directing. Each chord is assigned a word. These words can be lyrics or simply made-up words to designate the melody. For instance, in "When you wish upon a star," the *when* chord is an E and a G in the treble. The bass director will have two or three other notes to assign to the word *when*. Then the director forms each sign in rhythm and the bell ringer must remember which bell is to be played with each sign. This method of directing relies on each ringer remembering the signs. And the group must listen to each other in order to maintain the correct tempo.

Signing gives a multisensory approach to bell ringing. The ringer must first visually see the cue, cognitively remember which bell to play, physically ring the bell, and auditorily listen to the other ringers to play in rhythm. This is a proven, effective way of teaching any student who cannot read music how to become a performance-quality ringer. For each domain reinforces the next for total success.

As Nancy Tufts, author of *The Bell Ringers Handbook,* states:

When a child is cued, it is said to have a musical experience from contributing to a musical ensemble. But a child who responds without cue with a musical response demonstrates musicianship, understanding of one part relating to the whole—the final product.

Our ringers are literally set free enjoying the sounds of the choir and revelling in the awareness of their achievement. They use our cues as crutches, but they are the ones who have committed the song to memory.

The next step was to go "on the road for Jesus." When we first traveled, an autistic boy of about eighteen accompanied us. Phil had an uncanny gift of musical ability. He could tune the strings on his guitar, holding it to his ear to get the exact pitch. Then he would casually strum the most beautiful chords I had ever heard. Added to this was the gift of his strong young voice, singing clearly and distinctly, always in the right key.

Phil was a welcome addition to our choir. While he played, "You light up my life," the bell ringers signed as they stood behind their tables. It was a breathtaking experience. A heart-wrenching moment was when he sang Dallas Holm's song,

Why did you love me, Jesus?
How did you know my name?
Why did you save me, Jesus?
Oh, I'll never know, oh I'll never know.

In addition to his musical skill, Phil was quite unpredictable. Once we received an invitation to play our bells at a Lord and Taylor's department store in Pennsylvania. Before our concert we were scheduled to have breakfast with Santa.

The kids were excited. After breakfast, Santa came ho-ho-hoing into the room where we were eating and seated himself in a big chair up in front of everybody.

After the clapping died away, and the squeals of glee had subsided, Phil bounced out of his seat and seated himself right on Santa's lap. By that time Phil was nineteen-years old, almost six feet tall, of stocky build—not the average-sized candidate for sitting on poor Santa.

Phil was quite anxious to tell Santa what he wanted for Christmas, and there was no telling what Santa was thinking. Phil promptly whipped out of his pocket a folded-up piece of paper: his list for Santa Claus. In a high-pitched voice, loud and clear, he proceeded to read aloud:

THINGS I WANT FOR CHRISTMAS:

1. An American Express card (for travel)
2. Some American Express traveler checks
3. An airplane trip to Disney World
4. Two Beethoven symphonies
5. A Peter, Paul and Mary record

And on and on he rattled in his excited voice, his list endless. When Phil finished, he looked expectantly at Santa.

"Well?"

Santa regained his senses and managed to mumble, "I'll see what I can do."

I could imagine that under his whiskers his face was as white as his beard.

We had a small bus at Melmark that was used for field trips and it doubled as a means of transportation when the Joybells performed concerts for local audiences. Then the urge to travel hit us. We decided that we would go as far south as North Carolina for our first long-distance trek, back in 1981.

We wrote churches along our route and asked if they would be willing to let us present a concert in return for bed and breakfast and a light supper upon arrival. They responded, some warily, some enthusiastically.

Fortunately the bass director of the Joybells could drive our small bus. There was a wheelchair lift on it, which we did not need, but that was exactly the right spot to stack our bell choir tables, our dufflebags, and our bells. (There was no other storage space.) A small rod spanned the space on which we hung fresh blouses for our costumes.

The pile reached almost to the ceiling and on the very top, we piled our raincoats. This was a mistake, because they were slippery and slithered to the floor so very often, it got to be a family joke. Then we strapped everything back with black rubber straps as best we could. But each time the bus made a sharp turn, the huge mountain of luggage and gear shifted and started to fall.

Miss Ann and I sat opposite this pileup so that we could catch it in time. We often rode for hours with both feet planted firmly on the bell tables across the aisle. This was not too comfortable a position to assume for an extended period of time, so we took turns.

Fourteen hundred miles later, we received such a hearty welcome home that it was as if we were a team of astronauts, returning from outer space. That was just the beginning of our travels. We knew we needed a bigger bus. But buses were expensive and we had little hope of that item ever being considered a necessary plant fund item.

One day a director of a foundation came to visit. We talked about Melmark's needs, telling him of our remaining mortgages, which amounted to almost $300,000. Saying nothing, he jotted the figures down in his notebook. Then he asked whether or not we had any other pressing needs.

Paul looked at me and spoke up. I knew what he was going to say and I admired him for his courage. But I just knew it wouldn't work, for we had had many long talks about this need. My heart was in my mouth.

"Well, sir," Paul cleared his throat, "we need a new bus to carry our handbell choir so that they can go on tour. I think our choir can do much to erase some of the stigma that goes hand-in-hand with many mentally-handicapped persons. Their musical capabilities give dignity and worth to these special young people."

"And what would you think the cost of such a bus would be?"

"I imagine it would be in the neighborhood of $90,000."

Again, the scribbling of notes.

"Do you have other needs?"

I had grave misgivings at the prospect of ever getting that much money. Paul mentioned a need for two wheelchair vans with lifts. There was an agreeable nod of the head.

When he left, Paul and I looked at each other, wondering if we'd ruined our chances for receiving any money at all by mentioning so many needs.

Days later, there arrived a letter from that foundation. In it there was not only enough money to pay for a new bus, but enough to completely wipe out all our remaining debt! We could hardly believe it.

So we ordered the bus of our dreams. And how often since then we have given thanks to God for our beautiful new air-conditioned Blue Bird bus, complete with stereo tape deck, tilting seats, and even a breakfast nook where we prepared many a lunch while underway. Cupboards and sufficient storage space made us all feel like millionaires. And toilet facilities on board, clean and convenient, were there when needed.

How good our God is!

# 16

The alarm sounded at 5:00 A.M. Grateful that I had set the coffeepot on the timer, I shuffled out to the kitchen and poured two mugs, one for me and one for Melissa. She was still in her bedroom, burrowed under the blankets.

When I tapped her on the shoulder, she sat straight up, gave me a big grin, and reached for her coffee mug.

"Bell choir, Mommie! Bell choir!"

The phone rang. My secretary, Jean, who doubled as our bell choir bus driver, called dutifully on the phone to say that Hurricane Gloria was still out in the ocean twirling around, and she thought we would be at least one day ahead of it. Not to worry!

Jean, a single parent raising four beautiful daughters, was always enthusiastic and eager to start out on another adventure with our choir. No two tours were ever alike and this one already had the earmarks of winning a place in our diaries.

The sky was gray-streaked and foreboding. Perhaps it was only because of the "hurricane hype," but there was a tight little knot of fear in my stomach.

Paul, roused by the phone, pulled himself out of bed sleepily, downed a cup of coffee, and toted our suitcases, bus bags, and hanging costumes out to the car. When we got to Melmark, the orange and white bus was warming up. The kids greeted us with wild abandon.

Everyone was there, except our talented young music therapist, Celia. Miss Ann sat at the little breakfast nook in the back of our Blue Bird bus, fretting and scolding herself for not phoning Celia to make sure she was awake.

Miss Ann, a housemother at Melmark, accompanied our group to each concert. She was a large woman, carrying her considerable weight easily. Her round face, framed by short blondish hair, took on the look of an army drill sergeant at those times when she assumed effortless command of whatever situation she found herself in. Her empty threats were never carried to completion, but to her listeners they bore the full weight of impending and imminent doom. Her ample bosom was a haven to all in the time of stress. To me, she was psychological ballast, as we traveled far and wide from our Melmark nest.

In the midst of the drizzle, Celia banged loudly on the door of the bus. Greeting us with a big smile, she carried her suitcases to the back of the bus, her buttons unbuttoned, shoe laces untied, name tags sticking out at the back of her neck.

"Hey, I'm so sorry—my alarm didn't go off! You wouldn't believe how I hurried. Will we get there in time?" Breathlessly, her apologies poured out.

Miss Ann reassured her and handed her a cup of coffee, as she hung up Celia's costume and raincoat in the back.

"Everyone ready now?" Paul asked.

He walked to the front of the bus and prayed for safety and that we would be a blessing wherever we went. And so we were on our way. King's College was first on the agenda. We arrived at their gymnasium in plenty of time to set up for chapel.

The reaction of the student body was overwhelming. The choir was elated. And when red-haired Janet Benson sang her solo, "My Father's Eyes," many students were reduced to tears. A standing ovation was the climax of our concert, after which we ate lunch in the cafeteria and checked with the weather station again.

"Latest reports have Hurricane Gloria 350 miles south of Nags Head, North Carolina."

Despite the wind and the rain, we were not in danger. And the nasty weather was to be expected. We wended our way to Groton, Connecticut, where an evening church concert was scheduled at the Bible Chapel.

Setting up our bells that evening in the church, we watched the worried leader as he kept coming in, then disappearing. He'd talk a little about the weather and then apologize for what he thought would be light attendance that evening.

"You know how it is with church folk; they get all riled up about a hurricane, even though it's still out to sea."

The bounteous evening meal went down with little complaining and the brave souls that ventured out that wet evening were bound together by a feeling of anticipation that something momentous was about to happen.

After the concert, two by two, we were escorted by our sponsors to their homes. Melissa and I paired up. Every home was different, of course, and it was always interesting to watch Melissa sort out her apprehensions. She would only tolerate one dog, our big Great Pyrenees, and hated all cats instantly, without exception, on sight.

So, on this particular evening, Melissa had a few problems to deal with. There was a huge fuzzy cat squatting in the driveway. Sensing her fear, our sponsors hastened to assure her of the cat's gentle disposition, but Melissa was not convinced.

Unfortunately, the cat followed us as we went inside with our luggage. Melissa gave a sharp cry of protest as the cat brushed against her leg. They put the cat out, and then, from the direction of the back yard, a dog barked loudly.

Melissa's fright was easy to detect. She hid nothing. Her transparent reactions were always visible for everyone to see. This had initially caused me some embarrassment, but I found I could not possibly teach her all the polite little cover-ups that most people use to camouflage their real feelings.

At the sound of the dog, Melissa wanted one thing—to get out of there—so I took her upstairs. She bathed and was in bed, under the covers, in record time.

The eleven o'clock news confirmed my worst suspicions. The hurricane was going to come in at Groton—sometime the next afternoon!

When morning arrived, the blowing trees and light drizzle had all the telltale signs of the impending "blow." We listened to the weather station on TV while eating breakfast. But, after a few minutes of the "very latest about Gloria," the screen went blank. We tried to get the weather station on the phone, but the lines were busy.

Paul had flown down to see our Dallas family in Texas, so it was up to me to make a wise decision. I called Jean. She was cheery and bubbly, as usual.

"Jean, we need to fill up with diesel before we leave. I will call my daughter in Massachusetts, and see what direction they think we should head."

Diane's husband, Ron, was home and he said he had just heard that the eye of the storm was due to go right through the area where they lived. "Even though we'd love it, Mom, I don't think you should come this way. We're getting strong winds already. Now you be careful about power lines that might come down. I heard on TV that Boston is virtually closed down. I think the best thing for you to do would be to head due north and west. We'll be praying for you."

When we got to the church, everybody was there. The wind was beginning to gust, but we saw other cars on the streets, so we took heart. I expected the worst, yet prayed for the best.

A dear little lady escorted our bus to a man who owned a gas station. He opened up the station just for us, so that we could fill our tanks, and then refused payment—an unexpected blessing!

As we headed for Hartford, Miss Ann took inventory of our little pantry cupboard. We had plenty of bread, peanut butter and jelly, and granola bars, apples, and yogurt in our cooler.

The kids began to mirror our anxiety and everyone in the bus needed some encouragement. Bill sat there covering his eyes with both his hands.

"Hey, Bill, take your hands away from your big blues. We need all the men we can get," Celia yelled animatedly from her copilot's seat. She put on a Bill Gaither tape and our spirits picked up as we all joined in singing the familiar songs.

Passing the Connecticut River, we noted that many small boats were anchored to ride out the impending storm. The wind was sporadic, gusting and fierce one minute, and dying away the next. The rain was pelting down steadily. Five lanes of traffic fed into two, and the congestion was terrible. We had no way of knowing whether or not our decision had been a wise one. Little did we know that we were in the direct path of Hurricane Gloria.

The kids spotted the familiar orange roof and we made for the welcome shelter of Howard Johnson's. Anxiety was high but at least we were off the road.

Outside the winds picked up in velocity. As we settled into our five rooms, I noted with dismay that the beds had not been changed. I spotted some clean linens on a cart down the hall and asked the maids if we could have enough sets of bedding to make up our own beds. They weren't thinking about linens but were very apprehensively glancing out the window, muttering about having to get home before the hurricane hit.

We all trooped down to the ice machine and filled our buckets so that we could keep our big cooler chilled. Back in the room, the electricity went off again. The emergency lights went on in the hallways, so our rooms were lit only by the light from the windows. We pulled open the drapes.

Someone suggested that we phone the church where we were to perform next. But the phones were down as well. Even the restaurant had closed, so we enjoyed more of Miss Ann's famous peanut butter and jelly sandwiches. As we munched, we listened to our portable radio. The weathermen were having a field day.

"Jim McDonald here, standing weather watch. The next two hours are going to tell a story around here. Hurricane Gloria is moving very rapidly northward now. We expect the winds to be the strongest in London County, anywhere from seventy-five to one hundred miles an hour. Now, for our list of cancellations. Everything that is not essential has been postponed. . . ."

Somehow, intimate details of the storm only heightened our fears—mine, in particular! It wasn't long before we heard that the storm had veered and was due to go right through Hartford, Connecticut.

We stood on the balcony watching the trees, hearing them crack, some falling and some managing to snap back and stand tall again, before bowing once more to the fierce winds. The parking lot was flooded all around our bus and on the highway there was not a car or truck in sight.

After two or three hours of wind and rain, we all decided to take a rest. Outside we noticed the sky beginning to get lighter. Then the sun came out. We all let out a healthy cheer. But perhaps this was the eye of the storm. Needing to stretch our legs and work off excess nervous energy, we decided to take a walk outside and get a look at the damage.

A hamburger place next door to us had their windows protected by wide strips of taping, but their big front window was all smashed in.

We spotted a small coffee-and-doughnut shop next door to the restaurant. A young man inside poked his head out the window and yelled, "Hey! Could you use some doughnuts?"

"We sure could!" I called back. Excitedly, we ran over to the window.

"We're not open and we don't know what to do with all these doughnuts and muffins. How about some milk, too?"

"Fantastic! We have sixteen in our group, twelve handicapped boys and girls and four adults. And nothing's open as far as I can see."

"Where you staying? Howard Johnson's? Listen lady, you better be real careful; this is a very bad area. Keep your doors doubly locked and don't go out walking at night!"

He loaded us down with four boxes of all varieties of doughnuts, three quarts of milk, bran muffins, huge cookies, and a big bag filled with chocolate brownies. We could hardly wait to show our loot to Miss Ann. We had a bountiful supper of yogurt, milk, doughnuts, and an apple. It was a "five loaves and two fishes" miracle!

It was getting darker by the moment. Back in our rooms it looked as though we were due to get a glimpse of the other side of Gloria as the hurricane passed by us.

Bath time was somewhat unusual that night. We only had one huge flashlight from the bus, and we took turns using it. When we had all finally bedded down, the electricity was still off.

Around midnight all the lights came on, blazing in our eyes. We almost jumped out of our beds. Then we all settled down to sleep again and I dreamed of the hot coffee we would be having the next morning to go with our delicious doughnuts.

The next morning all of Connecticut, it seemed, was lined up to eat breakfast at Howard Johnson's. When our group of sixteen got in line, there were stares and grumbling. After about fifteen minutes, I talked with the manager to see whether we could buy cartons of orange juice, boxes of cold cereal, and a few quarts of milk to take up to our rooms. He willingly obliged, seeing an amicable way of getting us out of the dining room.

And then it was back to our bus. It felt good to be underway again. The drone of the diesel engine was like music to our ears. The rest of the trip went without a hitch. But none of us will ever forget the excitement of Gloria.

And then there were the Lizzies, with whom we fell helplessly in love. Lizzie—with the laughing eyes, riding her two-wheeler around campus, running races with her friends, arms and legs in beautiful symmetry. Lizzie—ringing bells in the Joybell choir, eyes crinkling at the corners.

I don't suppose that we ever could have readied ourselves for that telephone call in the middle of the night. It was Lizzie's father. His voice was barely controlled as he told us that Lizzie had died in the recovery room after what should have been a routine cardiac corrective surgery.

I was stunned, crying out my disbelief. There were no words of comfort for me to give out; I was deep in the valley of my own tears. Lizzie was always by my side whenever our handbell choir went on tour. She had a habit of gently nudging me to ask if she could sit next to me, or hold my hand.

The week before she went into the hospital, we had a mountaintop experience playing for eighteen hundred people, all either directors or bell ringers, at Ithaca College. Their enthusiastic reaction left us all a little overwhelmed. And we had excitedly started to plan our October tour.

I wondered how the choir would react when they heard of Lizzie's death. They knew she hadn't even been sick. Most of them couldn't understand why she even had to go to the hospital.

I tried to explain to Melissa what had happened. Filled with apprehension that she would not understand, I began, "Let's pretend that this doll is Lizzie."

Melissa knew about Grandma Rix dying, but Grandma was old and sick. Lizzie was different. Melissa looked at me as I picked up her doll with the blue eyes that opened and shut. I very tenderly laid the doll flat on her bed and closed the eyes of the doll with my hand.

"Lizzie is not sleeping, Melissa. Lizzie went up to heaven and now she is going to live up there with Jesus. You won't see her in bell choir any more. She left her body behind, but Lizzie is all gone."

I knew I was mumbling inanities. So much for my explanations. Melissa turned away from me without a word, picked up her doll, and walked away. I felt she had not understood a single word. When I called her for dinner later that day, she walked into the dining room with her doll stretched out on her tennis racket. Before she seated herself at the table, she very gently placed it on a chair. Neither Paul nor I could speak.

Three days later, there was an open casket memorial service in memory of Lizzie. When we walked into the funeral home, Melissa's eyes were filled with quiet wonder. We stood and looked at Lizzie, who somehow was not our Lizzie any more. Tears welled up, and Melissa grabbed my hand.

When the rest of the bell choir walked in, they stood before the open casket, looking in solemn disbelief at their friend lying so quietly in her beautiful satin bed. Then, they turned to each other and stood, not moving, but crying quietly and hugging one another. I thought my heart would burst.

The minister spoke of Lizzie racing around the portals of heaven, talking with Jesus, and waiting and watching until her heavenly family was united once more. And we all remembered the precious promises that God gives those of us who believe in him. There is life eternal for those who believe. Our hearts nodded a silent assent, for Lizzie knew and loved Jesus.

On the way home, one of the girls told me that she had touched Lizzie's hand. "It was cold, Mommie Krentel, and kind of hard."

"I know," I said.

"I whispered to Lizzie," Janet continued. "Oh, I know she couldn't hear me, but I told her not to worry because soon I was going to be in heaven, too."

And if I needed any further affirmation that they truly understood where their Lizzie was, it came about a month later at bell choir rehearsal. We had been going over a particularly difficult piece of music. Bill had been assigned to ring Lizzie's bells in this piece. He was really concentrating—and missing his cues. Suddenly, it all seemed to come together. He tilted his head back and raised both his bells heavenward.

"I got it, Lizzie, I remembered!" he exulted.

# 17

It was the hot, hot month of July. Our Texas and Florida families had flown up or driven by car to the Brookhouse, where we all would be together again for two glorious days of an old-fashioned family reunion.

Saturday dawned bright and beautiful, appropriate weather for such a celebration. It was fun-and-games day from breakfast to midnight snack. Physical from the onset, there were games of baseball, plenty of good-natured rough-housing, playing in the brook, swimming in Melmark's outdoor pool, and hard-fought games of tennis. The heads of families were tired out long before their offspring. We watched slides, drank coffee, traded jokes, and enjoyed one another's company.

I worried a bit about Sunday. How would all twenty-one of us ever get ready for church on time? Dave, our oldest son, and minister of a large church in Texas, suggested that we hold our own family church in the front living room.

Steve and Dave, our two minister sons, put their heads together and decided that it would be very meaningful also to have a communion service. We gathered in the living room on Sunday morning, the younger ones sitting on the floor. Steve led in the singing of favorite hymns and children's choruses. They loved every minute and would have gone on singing the rest of the day. Things were rolling on smoothly despite my forebodings.

Then David spoke very seriously: "Now, we are going to remember the death of Jesus by having a communion service."

I wondered if the children would behave; there certainly were some young ones present.

"Let's talk for a bit about what communion means."

Hands waved wildly in the air and childish voices offered

121

their simple explanations: "Not forgetting Jesus . . . I know, I know. The bread stands for his body when he dies on the cross . . . and the grape juice is for his blood. . . ." All the answers were right on target! David smiled.

"Now, before we have our communion service, I think we should have a little time of sharing and testimony. This is what I want each one of you to do." His voice was quiet, and the room was just as quiet as they waited to hear what Uncle Dave was going to say.

"Everyone is to get up and walk very quietly all around Nanna's house. Look for an object, some little thing that will help you tell how you feel about Jesus, maybe something he has done for you, or just something that will remind you to tell us what you know about him."

"Then," he continued, "when you find something, just pick it up and take it with you quietly back to where you are sitting. This is real serious. Just don't take Nanna's good china."

They all got up, as though they had been commissioned to find the Holy Grail. Nobody looked at anyone. Each seemed to take his lead from Uncle Dave, who very solemnly stood up and walked, with his hands behind his back, through the kitchen and out to the porch.

Benji found a ruler. I watched as he tucked it out of sight behind his back. Julie found a flashlight and hid it so Benji wouldn't see. Melissa got her Bible from her room and held it up proudly for me to see before she sat on it with the air of a conspirator. Alison found a hand mirror in the bedroom, and Laura spied one of my pet rocks.

Mission accomplished, all walked silently back to their seats. Even my ninety-year-old mother had something in her hands.

"We'll start with the oldest and work down to the youngest. Grandma, what do you have behind your back?"

Grandma held up a white tin cup. The enamel was chipped. "This used to be Grandpa's cup. He took it to college with him and he used to drink his coffee from it and later he kept change in it. He always said his cup was never completely empty, either of money or coffee." She brushed a tear from her eyes as she remembered God's faithful provision throughout their married life.

There was a yardstick, "So God could measure if we are growing or not"; a candle, "Jesus is the light of the world"; a Bible, "God's Word—we should read it every day."

Someone brought out a gladiola to symbolize new blossoms taking over when the old ones faded and dropped; no growth could take place unless the old ones fell off and died. There were two pennies, "That's what that poor lady put in God's offering plate"; an hour glass to remind us that our life is passing by and that we can never get back the time that passed; a notebook and a pen to remind us of God's book of life and names that he is writing down.

As each one spoke of his or her object, it was placed on our coffee table. I looked at them all through misty eyes and wondered what God would think of these small mementoes, spread out before his eyes, reminders of his love toward us and of his promises.

Then it was time for communion. Each family group was asked to sit in little clusters. The oldest child in each family was asked to come, one at a time. Steve pulled apart a big portion of French bread. Each one took it to his father, and the head of each household quietly broke it and gave a small piece to each member of his family. After giving thanks for the "body of Christ," the pewter mug, half-filled with grape juice, was passed around. Each one took a sip.

Even the youngest realized that this was very serious and a time of worship. There was no laughing, just the sweetness of a shared experience. I smiled to myself at my needless worrying. Why was it I felt that only the traditional ways of formal worship were the safest? Here we had shared a unique and intimate togetherness, a family memory to tuck away and hold fast.

It was the summer of '86, and it was raining. We had rented two cottages in New Hampshire at Lake Winnipesaukee. There were two cottages, four families, eight grandchildren, and one old wooden Century inboard. The boat was over at the marina in the bay, getting repaired. Paul telephoned with the discouraging news that the boat simply would not start and that a man had promised to help him.

The skis were lined up on the dock waiting for a miracle. Surely Pop-pop would come soon, roaring around the cove, motor at full throttle. Kathy and Dave were planning to leave that very afternoon for Canada, and the prospect of even one chance to ski on the lake seemed dimmer and dimmer. But the rain did not prevent swimming, so the kids all jumped into the water whooping and hollering as someone got dunked.

Suddenly, their hilarity was broken into by the unmistakable sound of a healthy inboard rounding the bend. An uproarious cheer went up. Pop-pop was the hero, wet and sodden, but victorious. The rest of the afternoon was spent in, or rather on top of, the water, as adventurous ones zoomed by, showing off their acquired skills. Those who did not ski went skimming by on top of the water on the surf board.

Then the Canada contingent departed and there were only twelve of us left. That second week, the weather about-faced and decided to cooperate. There were seven caned rockers on the front screened porch, facing due west. Rocking became the favorite after-dinner treat, each of us enjoying the magnificent sunsets. Each night, through the trees standing tall at the lakeside, the sun set faithfully and splendidly. And as we settled down with that second cup of coffee, we tried to determine the precise time for that perfect sunset picture. Each one was better than the last, or so it seemed. And there was ample time for relaxed conversations.

One evening, it was especially quiet. The kids were all up at Ron and Dee's cottage playing Monopoly, Ruth and Dee were down at the laundromat, and Paul and I sat on the porch with Bob, rocking and talking . . . quietly, reflectively.

Sharing some of our concerns for the future of Melmark, Paul turned to Bob and asked, "Son, would you ever consider coming back to Melmark?"

"If this is what God wants for my life, Dad, I would be back at a moment's notice."

Nobody spoke. I could hardly believe my ears. Each one of us was on his own "what if" trip. I felt a big lump in my throat. The question had been on the tips of our tongues so many times.

"I am honored to think that you both might welcome me

back again. It would be like coming home, in a sense. All of this experience has been very valuable, not only for me, but even for Melmark." For Bob had been serving mentally-handicapped youngsters in Vineland, New Jersey at AIMS (American Institute of Mental Studies, the former Vineland Training School). He had acquired broad management skills assisting the administrator for the past seven years. AIMS, with a population of well over two hundred residents, was situated on eight hundred acres of New Jersey countryside.

I can't remember what else was said that evening, but Paul and I had peace in our hearts and a song of thanksgiving to God for the possibility of Bob returning to Melmark, sharing the future of our family project. We wondered how the next step would be revealed to us—and when the time would be right to take it.

September rolled around. Paul and I invited Bob and Ruth over for dinner, not even hinting at what we wanted to talk about with them. So it came as a surprise to both when Paul asked Bob when he might feel ready to come back home to Melmark.

"You know, Bob, Mom and I are not getting any younger. I'll be sixty-seven next year. I want to hand over the torch while I am running strong, while I am still able to lend that support and strength that God has accorded me."

Later, Bob told us that he really never needed the week that he asked us for to pray about it. He was truly ecstatic. And our board of directors was equally elated.

Soon after the first of October, Bob and Ruth came to Pennsylvania, temporarily moving in with us until a suitable location was ready. Scott Robert, their eldest son, was away at Stonybrook School on Long Island.

I will not soon forget the informal welcoming party at Melmark the first week that Bob was back. It was one of those spontaneous affairs, with a large sheet cake and gallons of punch served simply in our board room. The boys and girls and the staff that had known Bob trooped in to welcome him back. Some reached up and touched his beard, some shook his hand, but most gave him a hearty bear hug.

Then there was the one boy who made it three times through the line. Finally Bob said, "Lee, you must be hungry." Grinning from ear to ear, Lee nodded happily, blew his nose on a paper napkin with one hand, and grabbed another piece of cake on the way out.

We decided that we should officially welcome Bob home. So on June 28, 1987, families and friends gathered together in our gymnasium to welcome Bob. It was a gala affair.

Paul stood to his feet, and asked Bob to stand beside him. His eyes seemed teary, and I was afraid that he was too moved to even make a speech, but his voice was strong as he placed one hand on Bob's shoulder.

Today is a momentous day in our personal lives and in the life of Melmark. We have set aside this day to mark a special occasion, a time to recommit our trust and confidence in a new leader.

There is no mantle, Bob, no divining rod, no golden scepter to transfer to you, my son. Just these promises from God to undergird you today, tomorrow, and in the coming years.

When Moses handed the leadership of the Israelites over to Joshua, it was a solemn, serious time. Moses reminded Joshua of God's precious promises. Today I remind you, Bob, that these promises are for you as well.

"Just as I have been with Moses," God said, "I will be with you. I will not fail you, nor forsake you. Do not tremble or be dismayed, for the Lord your God is with you wherever you go."

Twenty-one years have passed since the founding of Melmark, and as I reflect on our beginnings and ponder all that has passed over the years and all that Melmark will face in the future, it challenges and defies even the most stouthearted of men.

Life has not been without its problems: unfounded accusations by those we call neighbors, attempts to hold to a steady course as we steer Melmark in the face of all the current ideologies, battling for parents who would not have their handicapped child move away from lifelong friends and a place he or she has called home for so many years.

To you parents we say, we have loved your children until we have ached from the loving, we have wept until our hearts can find no more tears, and we have laughed at times until we collapsed. And it has been good. For if we did not laugh, we would cry until our weeping ceased.

Looking back through all the ups and downs of Melmark living, I would not undo or erase one moment. God has been faithful and he will continue to be just that as we persevere in our incredible journey.

So today, without fear or misgivings, I welcome my son Bob as the second president of Melmark and take this opportunity to assure him that my prayers will undergird him as he carries high the torch of Melmark. Our sights will be even higher as, with his young strength and vigor, and undergirded by the unsurpassed cooperation of our dedicated management team, the challenges of the future will be met.

As for me and my plans for the future, I seem to have come full circle. I have moved my office, quite symbolically, to the second floor of Melmark, to the room that was occupied by our first five residents: the Orange Room! You will find me there, behind that door which now sports the more sophisticated sign: chairman!

It will delineate my new responsibilities as chairman of the board and chief executive officer of Melmark, for I have no plans for retirement at this time. I desire to undergird the strengths and assure the future goals of this home that love built.

I plan with my wife Miggy, and God's enabling, to raise sufficient scholarship funds to help those of our parents who are burdened by the constant financial drain of providing services for their handicapped youngsters. This, along with the capital goals of the Twentieth Anniversary Fund, will be our project. We will need your prayers.

Bob, I am trusting you with the future tomorrows of your sister Melissa and all of her friends at Melmark. My confidence is complete. May God richly bless you in all the coming years.

His voice broke as he gave Bob a bear hug. And there was not a dry eye in the audience.

That very afternoon my ninety-three-year-old mother went home to heaven.

*Two homecomings in one day, Lord. How will I be able to bear the happiness of one and the sorrow of the other?*

# 18

I do not know the exact date that Melissa decided to live with Paul and me. She had her little room in the Tower House where four of her friends lived, and she also had her own room in our house. Sometimes she would choose to come with us, and sometimes she would say, in response to my requests, "No, Mommie—Tower House!" And I would pretend to cry.

But now, for whatever reason, Melissa has decided to live with us. For the last six or seven years, we have celebrated life together. We are honored to have her, and I suspect we need her far more than she needs us.

For she has added a new dimension to our living. Each morning she wakes up happy, and delights in the routines that daily life brings. She goes off to school each morning and returns home again in the afternoon, ready to follow her familiar ritual. First, a diet soda, then Sesame Street and Mr. Rogers. Once that is over, she sets the table: three placemats, three forks, spoons, and knives, and the always present coffee cups. The clearing of the table and stacking the dishwasher are chores she participates in cheerfully. She gets much satisfaction from performing simple tasks.

What effect has living with Melissa, day after day, had on Paul and me? My mothering skills are certainly being refreshed. Now I must remember all over again what I used to do so offhandedly in my earlier years. Back to supervising of showers, shaving of legs, shampooing of hair . . . the frequently-repeated lessons on how to properly brush teeth and comb hair, how to choose the right clothes for the weather and the occasion. I am constantly aware that she continues to need overseeing—and probably always will.

The heartache of having a retarded child does not lessen as

time goes by. The dead-end dreams, the endless quest for miraculous light at the end of some tunnel, the nonreversible chromosomal damage—they are here to stay.

Melissa is, and always will be, mentally retarded. Nothing will ever change that.

But, in everything give thanks, for this is the will of God in Christ Jesus concerning you (1 Thessalonians 5:18).

*God's will? My twenty-three-year-old daughter still playing with Raggedy Ann and Andy? Barely able to write her first name or read a book? Speech that is difficult, if not impossible, to understand? Incapable of tying her own sneakers, or buttoning the small white buttons on her blouse? Unable to communicate the frustration that makes her cry hot, angry tears? This is where the hurt is. It's where all the Melissas in the world are, and we must accept that fact.*

Strangers to Melissa's world are often unwittingly callous in their reactions to retardation. Why is it that grown people in public places turn around and stare, young people gawk, and suddenly the shopping spree or dinner out turns into a nightmare? The struggle goes on. And I am certain that most of it is on my side.

*Why do I fight so to make her act and seem normal? Why do I squelch her out-of-tune voice in church? She looks at me reproachfully, as though I were trying to stifle her worship. And I guess I am, for it embarrasses me. I've discovered that I'm such a proud person.*

But Melissa is different. Her disarming take-me-as-you-find-me approach to everyone only enhances her different upside-down self. Sometimes, it catches people off guard. They don't expect her to have a temper or to have strong likes and dislikes, believing that these special children are supposed to be passive, always agreeable, accepting of everything and everybody.

And most of the time she is. But when she isn't, she has no disguises. What you see is what you get! Color Melissa honest.

Whenever I am out with Melissa, I am often distressingly aware that everything we do or say, the love we show to one another, the obedience she may or may not accord me, the impatience that ebbs and flows, is all up front and center. We are pitifully, nakedly, on stage. So I have developed the skin of an armadillo. I can silently accuse the curious stranger with a long stare, or I can flagrantly ignore the situation and put on an act, knowing that our every move is being watched but pretending that I am not aware. And slowly they come to realize that they were being impolite, that they did not realize they were staring, and they apologize, eyes downcast.

But, despite my inner churnings, the indomitable, unquenchable spirit of Melissa continues to shine. Melissa makes us laugh when we're crying, love when we're unloving, and slow down long enough to see once again the humor in life. Through her unquestioning eyes, her mercurial forgiveness, her dependable and loving response, her unswerving loyalty, I am brought up short. The inner seething stops.

Melissa is outrageously happy and blissfully uninhibited. Her freedom to be her own self leaves me cheering on the sidelines—and envious that I do not enjoy the same liberty. She can pop into the board room after school with a brisk, "Hi, Daddy," drape her coat over the nearest chair, smile at everyone there, and be blissfully unaware that she has interrupted business. Her mission: money from Daddy to feed the soda machine, and then, she is blithely on her way home. Why, indeed, should I try to shape her to fit my mold, or the world's?

Melissa plays English handbells in a choir of twelve bell ringers. She has responsibility for five different bells, sharps and flats, and plays in time and with perfect rhythm—on cue! She does not give consistent eye contact, but tunes in by auditory means. In spite of this, she manages to play correctly almost all of the time, and is one of our better bell ringers.

She is very impatient, however, when we are learning a new song, and we can always depend on her to get irritated when someone makes a mistake and we must go back again and repeat the measure.

Melissa sings loudly off key in a strained vibrato, wavering between two notes. It is almost as if she were thinking, "I know the exact note is somewhere around here, so I'll try two at once." But does it really matter if the cadence she marches to is out of our earshot? Her parade throughout life is none the less triumphant, free, and glorious. And it is uniquely hers. She is free to be Melissa.

I have decided that I will always need a Melissa in my life. It's a humbling experience and one that keeps me from soaring out of sight. God knew I needed an anchor. And Melissa is just the right catalyst for our little family.

In spite of her inability to talk coherently, she is aware of exactly what is going on at any particular time. Her understanding is often unnerving. One Sunday, driving home after church, Paul and I had gotten bogged down in one of those petty little "nothing" quarrels. Melissa sat on the back seat and withdrew in her own silence.

Once inside the house, Paul stalked off to the bedroom and slammed the door resoundingly. Melissa and I stood there in the center hall and looked at one another. I dropped my handbag dispiritedly to the floor. Melissa folded her arms across her chest and said one word, "Daddeee!" followed by a pursing of her lips.

She was obviously convinced her Daddy was at fault, and I did not try to dissuade her. The humor of the situation began to bubble up. I looked at her with the air of a conspirator, and shrugged my shoulders.

"What are we going to do, Melissa?"

Melissa looked at the closed door and tiptoed toward it. Then she gave the door a quick staccato tap; there was no answer. She put her hand on the knob, looked at me for approval, then turned it and walked in our bedroom. Paul was just standing there.

Melissa grabbed both of his hands and pulled, literally yanking her father out of the bedroom over to where I was standing. The three of us stood there together in a little circle of her own making. Then she took one of my hands and placed it in Paul's big hand. Leaning her head against first one then the other of us, she lifted her face up toward us for our kisses. We had no choice. We all ended up in a tight little cluster of love, trading kisses and hugs indiscriminately, 'round and 'round.

Melissa has often assumed this role of peacemaker.

It's difficult to believe that Melissa is now twenty-three. She can tie her laces, button up even the smallest button. But she still writes only her first name, and in a scrawling print which wanders all over an eight-by-eleven piece of paper. She has no reading skills at all. Does this discourage me? I think not. I feel that it makes me a bit more understanding of those boys and girls who cannot, and do not, climb beyond some plateau, at whatever level it might be.

Bob has so often said to me, "Mom, if Melissa could talk plainly and read and write, would you be as sympathetic to those other hurting parents?"

And, honestly, I know he's right!

*I might be reduced to bragging. And what right do I have, anyway, to brag about something over which I have no control?*

Paul and I went shopping last Saturday at the King of Prussia Mall. We felt we just had to take time to get away, if only for a little bit. Lately it seems that I see my husband coming home from work, his shoulders sagging and the sparkle in his eyes gone. I catch myself thinking, "Is it really worth it all? Is our dream becoming a nightmare?"

When we arrived back home with our groceries and bird seed, we drove up to the Tower House, where Melissa stays when we are away, to pick her up for dinner. I was informed that she was over at the Rainbow Cottage with her house-mother and the rest of the girls.

Somewhat annoyed at having to make another stop, I bit my lip and said nothing. At Rainbow, I slipped on the ice and walked gingerly to the front door. A bevy of excited girls greeted me. The dining room tables had been shoved together and were topped with floured paper. There was a noisy, happy confusion in the cottage.

Some of the girls were garbed in aprons, enthusiastically making homemade pasta. There were smudges of flour on young faces and looks of anticipation on all. The aroma wafting from the kitchen was mouthwatering.

Standing there agog at all the hustle-bustle, my selfish impatience began to disappear. Melissa was sitting on the floor, an arm around one of her friends, watching TV. She looked disappointedly at me when I told her to find her jacket. While waiting for Melissa, I gravitated back toward the kitchen. An aunt of one of the house parents was supervising the project. She offered me a taste of their meatballs. I realized then how famished I was.

Not only a taste, but an entire meatball was consumed as I raved about her seasoning and hinted about her secret recipe. She not only shared her culinary prowess with me, but gave me seven meatballs to take home with me. I protested weakly.

As I left, Lori Beth, one of the Rainbow girls, said to me, "You can drop in to see us anytime, Mrs. Krentel." I smiled a happy grin, thanking her for the invitation.

As I left Rainbow, I thought about Melissa's day. She had been sledding earlier in the afternoon with the girls, loving every minute of it; then together they planned a pasta party.

*What is really happening behind the magic of these shared happenings? What is going on behind the scenes at Melmark? Melissa has a happy, fulfilling life—the kind of life she might not have had if there weren't Melmark.*

Putting Melissa to bed that night as I listened to her garbled evening prayers, I felt all my strength vanish. Taking a look at myself as I passed the mirror, I saw that my face looked drawn and haggard—I have become old!

*However did that happen? When was it that Paul and I became senior citizens? Am I being betrayed by my own body? This body is showing the signs of living more than I care to dignify by argument or flat denial.*

I smiled as I walked back to sit down on Melissa's bed, stroking her head and thinking of her precious Daddy.

*We need more than ever our times to be together, to be just Paul and Miggy again. To me Paul will always be the "young boy" that I fell in love with.*

I love that playing-hooky feeling that swept over us recently, as we got in the car and just headed off, away from Melmark. Paul pulled off to one side of the road, after five or so minutes, we folded back the rag top on our convertible, and, with a grin, he turned up the volume on our Dixieland jazz tape. The corners of his mouth went up and we shared a we-really-have-escaped look as we headed down the road. No destination, just going somewhere together!

*I still feel like an eighteen-year-old but the real me is imprisoned inside this sixty-six-year-old "ruined body." I am experiencing firsthand "the quiet endless tragedy that there was never a girl born who ever grew older than eighteen in her heart, no matter what the merciless hours have done."*

Old! Nowhere is this brutal fact harder to encounter than in the world of the handicapped. Those who have known a handicapped child and watched as he or she grew older have cried, as I have, as their future is pondered.

In their world, there apparently are no middle years. A child today, a senior citizen tomorrow. But inside those outsized bodies is that inner core of childlike innocence and trusting faith.

Was it not easier to bear when he was a baby or she was a cute little toddler? Nobody expected them to act "age appropriate," to order their own cheeseburgers, french fries, and soda, to stop drooling, quit gawking, and, for goodness sake, close your mouth when it's full of food. Nobody expected them to play with age-appropriate toys. "Throw away your Raggedy Ann, Melissa!"

What would they say to us, these childish minds in grown-up bodies?

> Walk a little slower, please! Wait for me to catch up. I am trying to follow, but I can't move as fast as you can. Please don't shout at me; I can hear your voice, but I don't always understand your words. Won't you be a little patient with me, please? What do I want? What do I need? I think I need to touch a handful of cool water. I need to pet something warm and soft and alive. I need to feel the hot sun on my back. I would like to walk with you through a puddle and splash both my feet. I need to have you sing to me, a happy song. Take my hand and dance with me.

Nobody heard our little talk by the bedside, Melissa. The hour is late, and you are fast asleep, and I—I am very tired.

Goodnight, my Melissa!

# Epilogue

I think that I have finally come to realize that a fitting climax for the end of this book is not now, nor will it ever be, able to be written. For life is going on at a rapid pace, and new and startling events are around each bend of the road. When indeed may I call the book finished? Will it ever be over? It seems to be a neverending story.

And there are stories which I must not tell, for fear of exposing someone else's private world. There are stories of despair that are too hurtful even to try to paint with words. And there are stories in the making . . . just waiting for the passage of time.

Philosophically, we are cutting against the grain of current ideologies which well might jeopardize all the Melmarks of today. There is but one answer, they say, one viable alternative, and they hold high the banner of "community living arrangements." CLA's often consist of three or four mentally handicapped persons living in a group home, situated in various neighborhoods.

To these crusaders it is the only solution, no matter how appropriate the situation, how stable the environment, how cost effective to the taxpayer. No matter to them whether parents, or the handicapped themselves, approve this change; the battle for the handicapped goes on.

And the handicapped themselves sit like helpless pawns in a chess game where politicos flex their muscles and moves are made without reason, without heart, in blind obeisance to some far-off drummer who thinks he knows the correct rhythm. The pawns are powerless, voiceless, easy to sacrifice. It is a game of life played on a cardboard table.

County after county continually send caseworkers to Melmark to view their clients, who now have become case numbers, in an attempt to fill those empty slots in a group home somewhere—anywhere.

And suddenly they are the experts at knowing what is best, and we, after a lifetime of living and interacting with these "clients," are classified as resistant to change, unwilling to move with the times because of our "vested interest."

All too often we see, almost as a ripple effect, the precious skills acquired by these retarded persons forfeited, as new surroundings impact their self-assurance, and a changing milieu is substituted for stable home environments such as Melmark. In the shuffle, the trust and confidence of the handicapped are sacrificed on the altar of change. It is good to remember that change is not always progress.

The community—is it ready? Will it ever be completely welcoming of these persons who lack so much? Who lack the ability to behave in a consistently socially acceptable manner? The ability to hold a non-supported job in the market place? The ability to travel and commute independently? The ability to verbalize and communicate needs and wants? The ability to cope with the daily stresses of "normal" living?

Do we need newspaper headlines to remind us of the zoning struggles, the neighborhood battles to exclude, the stigma and bias that go hand in hand with mental retardation?

These current issues are emotionally and physically draining. Some of the joy has gone, as we continue this costly battle for what we believe in. And I am not certain how long we will be able to continue.

Oh, the seesaw emotions we encounter daily in our Melmark world: the hope, the despair, the laughing, the crying. Each day is packed full. And sometimes there is just plenty of the ho-hum repetition of tasks that were part of yesterday, too.

So, for now, I think I will simply sit here and ponder. I will reflect on the lives of our own family and the effect that Melissa's life has had on each one of us.

It was Browning who described the two kinds of sorrow that man must endure in this life. One he called "escapable," and the other "inescapable." The escapable sorrow occurs when death strikes. It is swift, final, and irrevocable. The door is closed; the painful agony dissipates. As the days melt into months there is a welcome blurring of the memory, the soothing balm of healing. There is an escape. That was Martha!

The inescapable sorrow is that which must be faced when a crippling defect in body or mind occurs. It is much like a stone which is thrown into a pond. The placid waters part to receive the stone and then flow back together as the stone sinks slowly to the bottom of the pond. The waters are serene to the casual onlooker but the stone is still there and there it remains, buried and deep. An inescapable sorrow must be accepted and made friends with—for there is no escape. That is Melissa!

She has changed us . . . each one. I sometimes wonder whether or not my initial question is relevant now: "Will we end up devoting ourselves to our handicapped baby to the exclusion of our other children?" Or was it prophetic? I do not know. Melmark, a direct outgrowth of our Melissa-love, is a demanding mistress.

So, Melissa, if I were to write a legacy for you, I would leave to you the priceless gift of friendship: someone to laugh with you when you're silly, comfort you when you're teary, share a meal with you when you're hungry. I would leave to you a sheltered environment for as long as you need it.

It is funny, Melissa, I always think that Daddy and I will be the ones to leave you behind, for we are so very much older than you. And when that moment occurs and we must leave you, I know your heart will be sad. You will be bewildered and full of wonder, but it will only be for a while. You will get over it; you will laugh and giggle again without us, for you are far more flexible than we are. You will miss us, I am sure, but you have so many happy things to crowd into your life, that you will recover.

But listen, child of our hearts, if you leave for heaven before Daddy and I do, I know we have the assurance that you'd be up there waiting for us. But who would fill our emptiness, our sadness? Even now, I can hardly bear the writing of it, for what would we ever do without you? How essential you are to our everyday happiness! Can it be that after twenty-three years of loving, there is no lessening?

Little did Daddy and I dream when God allowed you to be

born to our family that he would simultaneously entrust us with this fulltime undertaking: Melmark. So much, from so little! God used us to pour out his love for you and your friends. How we thank him for entrusting us with an inescapable sorrow: Melissa!

Melmark is alive and well. God has blessed our efforts. He has exchanged our weakness for his strength, our shortsightedness for his vision, and he has used you, Melissa, our retarded daughter, as the catalyst to propel our energies toward helping to create something shining and beautiful: the home that love built.

Down syndrome occurs when a child is born with an extra chromosome in its genetic makeup. People normally have forty-six chromosomes within their cells that provide the information needed by the cells to grow and thrive. When reproduction occurs, chromosomes in sex cells split off into groups of twenty-three, containing genetic information from each parent. When the female's ovum is fertilized by the male's sperm, the twenty-three chromosomes from each parent unite, putting together forty-six chromosomes containing genetic information.

In Down syndrome, something happens in the chromosome division process that occurs before fertilization. Instead of splitting apart normally, two of the Number Twenty-one chromosomes stick together.

About three-fourths of the time this happens to the female ovum, but one-fourth of the time it occurs in the male sperm. The result is that when sperm meets ovum, there are three Number Twenty-one chromosomes in the mix instead of two, and the resulting individual has forty-seven instead of forty-six chromosomes.

The imbalance often results in spontaneous abortion, but if the fetus develops and is delivered the child experiences abnormalities such as mental retardation, retarded growth, and poor muscle tone. Physical characteristics include a small flat nose, slanting eyes, a protruding lower lip, and small hands and feet.

What causes the chromosomes' stickiness or "nondisjunction," as it is called by the physicians, is not understood. Doctors do know that the older a parent, the greater the risk of this occurring.

DR. GEORGE F. SMITH
CHAIRMAN OF THE RESEARCH COMMITTEE
NATIONAL DOWN SYNDROME SOCIETY
with Paul Feldman and
Dr. Gregory I. Smith

The Melmark Home Inc. is a nonprofit facility licensed by the Pennsylvania Department of Public Welfare for the care and training of the mentally retarded. Melmark is a private enterprise and receives no federal or state grants. Melmark is wholly dependent on student fees and monthly contributions for operation and maintenance costs.

Melmark's residential program is designed to meet the needs of the profoundly, severely, and moderately mentally retarded as well as those with multiple physical handicaps.

The Melmark School is a private academic school licensed by the Department of Education for the special education of the brain damaged, mentally retarded, and physically handicapped student. Melmark's coeducational twelve-month curriculum serves 188 residents from preschool age through adulthood from over 19 states and several foreign countries.

Melmark accepts residents from infancy through adulthood, regardless of sex, race, creed, or ethnic origin, who are able to benefit from the special care, training, and education that are offered.

The overwhelming majority of Melmark's residents are severely or profoundly retarded, often with many accompanying physical limitations—a segment of the handicapped population that many private and public schools do not admit.

Contrary to prevalent theory, Melmark believes that the learning process does not stop at eighteen or twenty-one years of age. Thus, Melmark provides ongoing education for this age group. Learning for the adult retarded person ensures ongoing stimuli in a goal-oriented medium and helps to prevent the regression that so often occurs with the aging process.

Despite the financial burden incurred by a commitment to lifelong education, Melmark has pledged itself to protect the rights of its residents to learn all they can for as long as they can. Creative programs offer socially and emotionally enriching stimuli for progressive life enhancement.

Melmark offers approved therapeutic programs in adaptive physical training, speech, music, horticulture, dried-flower arranging, aquatic skills, and horsemanship at no extra cost to students. Opportunities to perform in a variety of cultural enrichment programs such as the touring handbell choir, Special Olympics, and theatrical productions are integral parts of Melmark's creative programs.

The Creative Workshop programs offer a wide variety of challenging choices for residents to participate in activities that foster a productive lifestyle. Dried-flower arranging, ceramics, gardening, landscaping, woodwork, stenciling, rug hooking, and food processing are all components of a therapeutic environment that is focused on the aging retarded.

Elective subjects such as weaving, music and movement, square dancing, team sports, slimnastics, and weight training are also offered where appropriate.

The therapeutic horsemanship program at Melmark can best be described on two levels: physical and psychological. Each student in the program receives a complete analysis of his needs and a specific program is designed. Most students come to Melmark either with physically handicapping limitations such as hemiplegia, spina bifida, cerebral palsy, etc., or they are presented as developmentally delayed, overweight, uncoordinated, and generally out of tune with their bodies.

When a physically-handicapped student has no use of or limited use of his legs, the horse provides the broad base for balance necessary for the student to gain control of his trunk, neck, head, etc. There is a high degree of similarity between the movement of the pelvic girdle of a walking person and the movement of a rider on a walking horse.

Melmark is recognized for its creative and unique contributions made in the performing arts. Residents are motivated to achieve skills necessary to reach performance quality in ballet, drama, interpretative dance, and handbell ringing in choir context. Through the excitement of audience response, growth and development of these skills have reached an astonishing level.

"The Nutcracker," a Christmas fantasy, with special lighting effects, elaborate costumes, sparkling dance routines, and expressive pantomime, is participated in by over eighty students. Each year, the students grasp more difficult sequences and the precise timing demanded by the choreography. Melmark's stage is kept busy throughout the year as well, with school presentations.

Dr. Cathy Crossland, of the University of North Carolina, states: "While the academic program constitutes the cornerstone of Melmark School, there is a comprehensive array of supportive therapeutic programs that operate on the campus. Each of these programs is uniquely tailored to enhance self-esteem, promote physical and emotional wellbeing, and advance self-sufficiency and independent living skills in those individuals for whom such skills are reasonable. One of my most vivid impressions of Melmark was the determination of the staff members to seek ways to involve even the lowest functioning individuals in meaningful activity in each program. The concept of task analysis—reducing a task to its lowest possible terms for learning purposes—is regularly implemented in the educational and therapeutic programs. A large number of the residents I saw at Melmark who were busily engaged in therapeutic activities would be labeled as non-functional in most other environments."

Visitors touring the Melmark campus are struck with the realization that being handicapped at Melmark is not considered a deterrent to continuous daily involvement in productive activities. Melmark's living and program areas bustle with activity. This attitude of providing creative challenges demonstrates the philosophy on which Melmark was founded more than twenty years ago.